SLEEP SOUNDLY EVERY NIGHT, FEEL FANTASTIC EVERY DAY

SLEEP SOUNDLY EVERY NIGHT, FEEL FANTASTIC EVERY DAY

A DOCTOR'S GUIDE TO SOLVING YOUR SLEEP PROBLEMS

Robert S. Rosenberg, DO, FCCP

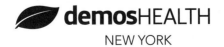

NEW YORK

Visit our website at www.demoshealth.com
ISBN: 978-1-936303-72-4
e-book ISBN: 978-1-617052-15-6

Acquisitions Editor: Julia Pastore
Compositor: diacriTech

Medical information provided by Demos Health, in the absence of a visit with a health care professional, must be considered as an educational service only. This book is not designed to replace a physician's independent judgment about the appropriateness or risks of a procedure or therapy for a given patient. Our purpose is to provide you with information that will help you make your own health care decisions.

The information and opinions provided here are believed to be accurate and sound, based on the best judgment available to the authors, editors, and publisher, but readers who fail to consult appropriate health authorities assume the risk of injuries. The publisher is not responsible for errors or omissions. The editors and publisher welcome any reader to report to the publisher any discrepancies or inaccuracies noticed.

Library of Congress Cataloging-in-Publication Data

Rosenberg, Robert S. (Robert Steven), 1948- author.
   Sleep soundly every night, feel fantastic every day : a doctor's guide to solving your sleep problems / Robert S. Rosenberg, DO, FCCP.
      pages cm
   Includes bibliographical references and index.
   ISBN 978-1-936303-72-4—ISBN 978-1-61705-215-6 (e-book)
1. Sleep—Popular works. 2. Sleep disorders—Popular works. I. Title.
   RA786.R67 2013
   616.8'498—dc23

Special discounts on bulk quantities of Demos Health books are available to corporations, professional associations, pharmaceutical companies, health care organizations, and other qualifying groups. For details, please contact:

Special Sales Department
Demos Medical Publishing, LLC
11 West 42nd Street, 15th Floor
New York, NY 10036
Phone: 800-532-8663 or 212-683-0072
Fax: 212-941-7842
E-mail: specialsales@demosmedpub.com

Printed in the United States of America by McNaughton & Gunn.
15 16 17 18 / 5 4 3

To Christine Feltman Rosenberg, my wife of thirty years, mother of my wonderful children, my executive producer, accomplished businesswoman, and occupational therapist. She inspired me to write this book and has been by my side every step of the way supporting my medical career, dreams, and now my mission to educate the world about sleep medicine.

Author's Note

The names and identifying characteristics of all patients have been changed to protect their privacy.

Contents

Introduction: Moving into Health Together   *xvii*
How to Use This Book   *xviii*

1   **Identifying Your Sleep Problem**   *1*
Sleep Disorder Checklist   *2*

**Part One: Sleep Foundations for Your
        Best Life**   *7*

2   **The Cornerstone of Health**   *8*
Sleep Stages and Cycles   *9*
The Effect of Too Little Sleep on Your Health   *12*
Fatigue and Brain Fog   *15*
Take the First Step and the Rest Falls into Place   *18*

3   **How to Get a Good Night's Sleep**   *19*
Identify Your Motivation   *19*
Create an Ideal Bedroom Environment   *21*
No Blue Lights at Night   *24*
Break Habits That Hinder Sleep   *24*
Habits to Aid Sleep   *25*
Dismiss a Worry or Dump an Attitude   *26*
Superb Sleep through Progressive Muscle
   Relaxation   *28*
What's Next?   *30*
Sleep Diary   *31*

Part Two: Impaired Sleep or Dyssomnias 35

4 **Restless Legs Syndrome 36**
What Is Restless Legs Syndrome (RLS)? *39*
Symptoms *41*
Treatment Options *41*
The Difference between RLS and Periodic
  Limb Movements *43*
Answers to Your Questions *43*
  Foot Pain at Night *44*
  RLS and Antidepressants *44*
  Why Do I Rub My Feet Together? *45*
  Are Gambling and RLS Related? *45*
  Relationship between RLS and Obsession *45*
  A New Medication and Leg Tingling *46*
  RLS Pain after New Medication *46*
  RLS Correlation to Attention Deficit
    Hyperactivity Disorder (ADHD) *47*
  RLS and Sleep Attacks *47*
  RLS and Exercise *48*
  RLS and Nonpharmacological Treatments *48*
  RLS or Fibromyalgia? *48*
  RLS and Varicose Veins *49*
Self-Check: Restless Legs Syndrome
  Checklist: URGE *49*

5 **Insomnia 51**
Primary Insomnia *52*
  Sleep Hygiene *56*
  Stimulus Control *56*
  Cognitive Restructuring *56*
  Symptoms *57*
Transient Insomnia *58*
Insomnia with Multiple Causal Factors *60*
Chronic Insomnia *63*
  Indications *64*
Why You Suffer from Insomnia *65*

Do You Have a Vulnerability to Insomnia? *66*
Insomnia and Women *66*
Treatment Options *67*
    Good Sleep Hygiene *67*
    Stimulus Control *68*
    Sleep Restriction *69*
    Cognitive Behavioral Therapy (CBT) *69*
    Cognitive Restructuring *69*
    Online Cognitive Behavioral Therapy *71*
    Release Tension and Relax Before
      Going to Bed *72*
    Medications *74*
Preparing for an Appointment with a
  Sleep Specialist *75*
Answers to Your Questions *76*
    Sleep Maintenance *76*
    Chronic Insomnia *76*
    Paradoxical Sleep *76*
    Drinking Coffee *77*
    Sleep Deprivation *77*
    Stress and Sleeping *77*
    Smoking *78*
    Husband Denying Insomnia *78*
    I've Tried Everything! *79*
    No Luck with Sleep Aids *79*
    Stop the Caffeine *80*
    Valium *80*
    Singulair *81*
Self-Check: Insomnia Severity Index *83*
    Scoring and Interpretation *83*

6 Circadian Rhythm Disorders *84*
Circadian Biology and a Normal
  Circadian Clock *85*
    Blue Light Pollution *86*
Circadian Rhythm Disorders *88*
    Jet Lag Disorder *88*

Symptoms Checklist *89*
Getting Help *90*
Delayed Sleep Phase Syndrome *93*
Symptoms *94*
Getting Help *94*
Advanced Sleep Phase Syndrome *96*
Free-Running Disorder *96*
Irregular Sleep–Wake Syndrome *98*
Shift Work Sleep Disorder *99*
Answers to Your Questions *101*
Effect of Light *101*
Getting Up in the Morning *101*
Irregular Sleep–Wake Disorder and
Alzheimer's *102*
Use of Seasonal Affective Disorder (SAD)
Lamp *102*
Jet Lag *103*
Shift Work Disorder *103*
Use of Sleep Aids *104*
Lack of Sleep Causing Illness? *105*
Difficulty Staying Awake on the Job *105*
Trouble Getting to Sleep After
Shift *105*
Medications to Stay Awake *106*
Staying Alert *106*
Impact of Age on Staying Awake *107*
Self-Check: Self-Assessment for Night Owls and
Morning Larks: Delayed Sleep-Phase Syndrome
versus Advanced Sleep-Phase Disorder *107*
Scoring *110*

7 No Sleeping with Apnea 111
Obstructive Sleep Apnea (OSA) *114*
How the Body Works on OSA *115*
Sleep Apnea, Hypertension, and Stroke *115*
This is Your Brain on Sleep Apnea *117*
Sleep Apnea and Diabetes *118*
Children and Sleep Apnea *119*

Symptoms   *120*
  Frequent Nighttime Urination   *121*
  Sexual Dysfunction   *121*
Treatment Options   *122*
  Continuous Positive Airway Pressure
    (CPAP)   *123*
  Mandibular Advancement Device
    (MAD)   *124*
  Positive Airway Pressure Nap
    (PAP-NAP)   *124*
  Hypoglossal Nerve Stimulator   *124*
  Weight Loss   *124*
  Uvulopalatopharyngoplasty   *125*
Central Sleep Apnea (CSA)   *125*
Answers to Your Questions   *127*
  Difference between CSA
    and OSA   *127*
  Teen's Breathing Pattern
    Is Apnea?   *128*
  Sleep Apnea and Children   *128*
  Sleep Apnea and Dementia   *129*
  Apnea and Blood Sugar   *130*
  CPAP   *130*
  Apnea and Epilepsy   *131*
  The Difference between CPAP and Adapto Servo
    Ventilation (ASV)   *132*
  What Is Complex Sleep Apnea?   *132*
  CSA and Methadone   *133*
  CPAP Caused CSA?   *133*
Self-Check: What Is Your Risk of OSA?: Stop
  Bang Questionnaire   *134*

Part Three: Parasomnias   *135*

  8 **Sleepwalking and Night Terrors   *137***
Sleepwalking   *137*
  Sleepwalking in Children   *138*
  Sleepwalking in Adults   *139*

NightTerrors   *142*
   Night Terrors in Children   *142*
   Night Terrors in Adults   *143*
Answers to Your Questions   *143*
   Lithium and Sleepwalking   *143*
   Sleepwalking and Genetics   *144*
   Driving in Sleep?   *144*
   Adult Sleepwalking?   *144*

9 Sexsomnia   146
Sexsomnia Behaviors   *147*
Causes   *149*
Are There Solutions?   *149*
Importance of Getting Help   *150*
Sexsomnia as a Defense   *152*
Answers to Your Questions   *154*
   Medications   *154*
   Stress   *154*

10 The Night Eaters   155
The Two Forms of Night Eating   *156*
Sleep-Related Eating Disorder (SRED)   *157*
   Treatment Options   *160*
Night Eating Syndrome (NES)   *160*
   Symptoms   *162*
   Treatment Options   *163*
Distinguishing SRED and NES   *163*
Answers to Your Questions   *164*
   Wife Eats Sugar   *164*
   Zolpidem   *165*
   What Can Be Done?   *165*
   I Am Awake When Eating At Night   *166*
Self-Check: Do You Have a Night-Eating
  Disorder?   *166*

**11 Do You Sleep, but Not Too Deeply? REM Sleep
Behavior Disorder   167**
Symptoms   *169*
  Symptom Checklist   *169*

The Importance of Rapid Eye Movement
  (REM) Sleep   *170*
    REM Benefits   170
    Lack of REM Sleep   173
  Treatment Options   *174*
  Answers to Your Questions   *175*
    Fighting for His Life   *175*
    Medication for REM Sleep Behavior Disorder
      (RSBD)   *175*
    Acting Out in Dreams   *176*
    Screaming and Thrashing   *177*
    I Moved to a Different Bedroom   *177*
    WatchPAT Device   *178*
    REM Sleep Abnormality?   *178*

Part Four: Sleep Disorders and Major Health Issues   *179*

12 **Sleep for Those with Post-Traumatic Stress Disorder**   *180*
  Gina's Story   *180*
  What Is Post-Traumatic Stress Disorder (PTSD)?   *183*
  PTSD Checklist   *187*
  Why It's Important to Resolve Sleep Disorders
    Related to PTSD   *188*
  Treating Sleep Apnea Improves PTSD
    Symptoms   *189*
  Insomnia and Short Sleep Duration in PTSD   *190*
  Nightmares   *192*
  Help for Sleep-Related PTSD Issues   *192*
  Answers to Your Questions   *193*
    Is Sleep Apnea Common?   *193*
    Vietnam Veteran Still Has Nightmares   *194*
    Sleep Study Okay?   *194*
    How Long Will Vietnam Nightmares
      Continue?   *194*
    Sertraline   *195*
    What Works?   *195*

Good Sleep, Bad Moods *196*
PTSD from Car Accident *196*

13 Sleep Disorders and ADHD *198*
Children, Sleep, and ADHD *199*
The Most Common Sleep Disorders Associated
with ADHD *202*
Daytime Sleepiness *202*
More Movement in Sleep: Restless Legs
Syndrome *202*
Sleep-Disordered Breathing, Sleep Apnea,
and Hypopnea *203*
Dr. Rosenberg's Checklist for Preschool and
School-Aged Children *205*
Adolescents and Adults *207*
Treatment Options *209*
Answers to Your Questions *210*
Sleep Apnea and ADHD *210*
Sleepiness *211*
Self-Check: Your Child's Sleep Habits *211*

Conclusion: Sleep Well *212*
Start Where You Are *212*
Use What You Have *213*
Do What You Can *214*

Appendices *215*
Better Sleep Quick Reference *217*
Attention Deficit Hyperactivity
Disorder Checklist *221*

Glossary *222*
Notes *231*
Acknowledgments *245*
Index *246*

Introduction: Moving into Health Together

Your life is a reflection of how you sleep, and how you sleep is a reflection of your life.

— DR. RAFAEL PELAYO

We need restorative sleep to survive and succeed. Without restorative sleep, we are out of sync with ourselves, each other, and with nature. Most likely you have picked up this book because you feel out of sync. You have trouble getting to sleep or staying asleep. You wake frequently in the middle of the night. You wake up tired. Or maybe it's your partner, child, or loved one who is keeping you up at night. Perhaps you are experiencing pain, fatigue, headaches, leg cramps, hyperactivity, chronic stress, or other symptoms you want to change or cure and suspect lack of sleep is playing a role. You know something is wrong and wonder if it's a common problem with a simple fix or something that requires professional help.

Sleep Soundly Every Night, Feel Fantastic Every Day can help you find the answers you are looking for. It will help you identify and understand your symptoms and guide you to the most likely problem or disorder. It also offers practical treatment solutions to help you get a good night's sleep right away and to determine if seeing a sleep expert is right for you. It will show you how to sleep deeply and experience the joy of a good night's rest.

We have come a long way in thinking of sleep as a passive state. Rather, we now know how active the sleep time is for the "neurobiological state," which regulates several functions of the body, including temperature, memory and learning consolidation, and metabolism. Disrupted sleep or a lack of sleep negatively affects these functions. Short-term sleep deprivation could result in

1. Decreased concentration
2. Irritability
3. Bad mood
4. Tremors
5. Hallucinations
6. Diminished immune function

Continued sleep deprivation results in an increase in metabolic rate, in appetite, and in body temperature, immune system failure, and decreased brain activity.

Lack of sleep dramatically impacts your health, ability to function, and well-being. Yet, Americans' sleep time over the last century has decreased by 20%. It is important to address problems immediately—and don't give up! A sleep solution *is* available for you and I will help you find it.

How to Use This Book

The self-test in chapter 1 will help you pinpoint your symptoms and direct you to the most useful chapters in this book to help you resolve them. *Everyone* should read Part One on the importance of sleep for your health and essentials for getting a good night's sleep. You may be inclined to skip ahead to the chapter on your particular problem, but I can't emphasize enough how important it is to start here. Once you learn about the negative long-term effects of poor sleep and how restorative sleep positively affects your physical health, executive thinking skills, clarity, and optimism in chapter 2, you will be eager to make the lifestyle changes outlined in the next chapter. Chapter 3 covers good sleep practices or good sleep hygiene. Since good sleep hygiene may resolve your issues or lessen their severity, make implementing these recommendations your first priority on your journey to good sleep.

The next three parts cover the most common sleep problems and disorders:

Part Two, Impaired Sleep, addresses three common sleep disorders that keep you from getting to sleep, staying asleep, or managing early morning awakenings. They are called dyssomnias and include:

- Restless legs syndrome, an intense, irresistible urge to move the legs in the evening.
- Insomnia, an inability to fall asleep or maintain sleep. It is the most prevalent sleep problem in America.
- Circadian rhythm disorders, when your internal sleep clock is out of sync because you travel or work a night shift.
- Sleep apnea, pauses in breathing or instances of shallow or infrequent breathing during sleep.

Part Three explains parasomnias, behaviors like walking, eating, or having sex that occur during sleep, including:

- Sleepwalking, an arousal disorder where the sleeper gets out of bed and walks.
- Sexsomnia, a disorder in which a person acts out sexual behavior while asleep.

- Night eating disorders, a persistent pattern of late-night binge eating.
- Rapid eye movement (REM) sleep behavior disorder, which is characterized by a lack of the usual sleep paralysis occurring during REM sleep. This allows the sleeper to act out any dreams.

Part Four presents two chapters in two areas where sleep disorders and psychiatric diagnoses overlap. Research has shown that it is essential to treat both. These include:

- Post-traumatic stress disorder (PTSD), an anxiety disorder that results from an experience or exposure to an extreme emotional trauma. Sleep disorders and PTSD have overlapping symptoms that affect each other.
- Attention deficit hyperactivity disorder (ADHD). The symptoms of ADHD and related sleep disorders present in similar ways, sometimes leading to a misdiagnosis of ADHD or a missed opportunity to alleviate the symptoms of ADHD by resolving sleep issues.

Each chapter on a specific sleep disorder includes a symptoms checklist, the latest treatment options, and answers to the most commonly asked questions about the disorder that I have received through my columns in *The Prescott Daily Courier* and the *Arizona Daily Sun,* and on my website, AnswersforSleep.com.

In the appendices, you will find additional resources to help you improve your sleep habits and sleep quality.

I have practiced medicine and provided treatment for thousands of patients for over 30 years. You are not the only one too tired to count sheep or move your body to go to the bathroom in the middle of the night. Far from it. The Centers for Disease Control estimates that 50 to 70 million Americans have sleep disorders. If you are one of those with a sleep problem, this book will show you how to improve the quality of your sleep. The quality of your sleep, in addition to how long you sleep, affects your health, and you *can* change it.

Let's get started.

- **Step One:** Answer the questions on the Sleep Disorder Checklist in the next chapter to identify your symptoms and areas of the book that will be of most help to you.
- **Step Two:** Read Part One. These two chapters provide an overview of the purpose, functions, and marvelous benefits of sleep and the basics of good sleep hygiene everyone should implement immediately.
- **Step Three:** Go directly to the appropriate chapters indicated by your answers to the Sleep Disorder Checklist. In these chapters, you'll find the most up-to-date information about your sleep issue, including likely causes, treatment options, and changes you can apply right away to resolve it.
- **Step Four:** Read the entire book and determine if your sleep issue overlaps with other symptoms, sleep disorders, or emotional patterns.

Identifying Your Sleep Problem

The most obvious sign of a sleep disorder is sleepiness during the day. Excessive sleepiness has varied causes and triggers that you need to know about if you intend to get to the root of your sleep issues. If you are sleepy, you may spend the next day wondering how to get a better night's sleep. If sleeping doesn't happen soon, you may become too sleepy to think about sleep. This circular pattern of being sleepy, worrying, and wanting to sleep is like not being able to see the forest for the trees. Your symptoms are right in front in you, and you are wandering through the forest and worrying. Wow, that drains your energy, doesn't it? Being proactive won't drain your energy; it will energize you. The first step is to identify your symptoms in the Sleep Disorder Checklist on page 2.

The questions will help you observe how you sleep so that you can change what isn't working and develop a new sleep plan. Consider whether each question is true for you. When you consider a question such as, *Do you wake up feeling like you barely slept at all?* you would answer "yes" if this happens at least two to three times a week. Think about how the issue is consistent or not, persistent or not, troubling or not.

Sleep Disorder Checklist

Question	✓ YES
Do you have trouble controlling your diabetes?	☐
Do you wake up feeling like you barely slept at all?	☐
When you get into bed at night, do you find it difficult to shut off your mind?	☐
Is your snoring so loud that it disturbs others?	☐
Do you have difficulty remembering recent events or names?	☐
Have you or a loved one been diagnosed with early dementia?	☐
Has your depression continued in spite of taking antidepressant medications?	☐
Does bedtime bring on feelings of anxiousness?	☐
Do you wake up in the early morning hours and find it difficult to go back to sleep?	☐
Do you suffer with morning headaches?	☐
Do you wake up in a sweat with your heart pounding and feeling anxious?	☐
Do you have difficulty staying awake when you are not engaged in an activity?	☐
Does it take you a long time to get going in the morning?	☐
Do you get up to urinate two or more times a night?	☐
Do you have an uncomfortable feeling in your extremities that keeps you from falling or staying asleep?	☐
Do recurrent nightmares disturb your sleep?	☐
Do you find signs of eating at night that you cannot recall?	☐

(continued)

Sleep Disorder Checklist

(continued)

Question	✓ YES
Do you act out your dreams, hurting yourself or others?	☐
Has your child been diagnosed with ADHD?	☐
Has a traumatic life experience or incident affected your sleep?	☐
Are you a night owl who has trouble getting up in the morning?	☐
Are you on more than two medications to control your blood pressure?	☐

Based on your answers, use the following chart to identify the chapters you should read first. Some symptoms overlap several problems and so multiple chapters are provided. Read all of the chapters suggested to help connect the dots about your sleep and create a complete sleep profile.

If you answered "yes" to:

Question	Go to Chapter
Do you have trouble controlling your diabetes?	7
Do you wake up feeling like you barely slept at all?	4, 5, 6, 7
When you get into bed at night, do you find it difficult to shut off your mind?	4, 5
Is your snoring so loud that it disturbs others?	7
Do you have difficulty remembering recent events or names?	4, 7
Have you or a loved one been diagnosed with early dementia?	7

Question	Go to Chapter
Has your depression continued in spite of taking antidepressant medications?	4, 7
Does bedtime bring on feelings of anxiousness?	4
Do you wake up in the early morning hours and find it difficult to go back to sleep?	4, 5, 6
Do you suffer with morning headaches?	7
Do you wake up in a sweat with your heart pounding and feeling anxious?	7, 11
Do you have difficulty staying awake when you are not engaged in an activity?	4, 7
Does it take you a long time to get going in the morning?	4, 5, 6
Do you get up to urinate two or more times a night?	7
Do you have an uncomfortable feeling in your extremities that keeps you from falling or staying asleep?	4
Do recurrent nightmares disturb your sleep?	11, 12
Do you find signs of eating at night that you cannot recall?	10
Do you act out your dreams of hurting yourself or others?	7, 11
Has your child been diagnosed with ADHD?	7, 13
Has a traumatic life experience or incident affected your sleep?	12
Are you a night owl who has trouble getting up in the morning?	6
Are you on more than two medications to control your blood pressure?	7

Now that you have a better sense of your symptoms, find out more about the benefits of resolving them and the best ways to do so. To understand how symptoms of a sleep disorder disrupt your life, the next chapter introduces the healthy kind of deep sleep you need and its outstanding benefits for mental, emotional, and physical health.

PART ONE

Sleep Foundations for Your Best Life

In Part One, you'll learn what constitutes healthy sleep and how restorative sleep works, the stages of sleep, and good sleep hygiene. A minimum of seven to nine hours of sleep improves significantly your ability to think clearly, maintain focus, and stay emotionally balanced.

2

The Cornerstone of Health

Silence is the sleep that nourishes wisdom.
—SIR FRANCIS BACON

The recent decade of sleep research has shown that sleep is one cornerstone of your health. Like water, nutrition, and exercise, sleep is vital to your quality of life, your ability to focus and think, and even your ability to empathetically relate to people. People need seven to nine hours of sleep *each* night to allow biological systems the time they need to regenerate energy, balance stress, and consolidate memory and learning. Sleeping deeply enables your body to balance and renew tired or stressed systems. You awaken from this type of sleep feeling refreshed, focused, and ready for your day. Yet, according to a National Sleep Foundation poll conducted in 2012, Americans average less than seven hours of sleep on weeknights. For the majority of people who do not sleep deeply, the brain and body experience alarming, debilitating symptoms.

Sleep Stages and Cycles

The two dimensions of sleep most important for you to know are *duration*, how long you can and need to sleep, and *depth*, your ability to reach and sustain uninterrupted deep sleep. You need to sleep long enough and deeply enough to give your body the time it needs to recharge, stabilize, and balance the internal functions. Think of what is required to recharge a dead car battery. First, you need a strong, uninterrupted charge that sparks the battery to regenerate power. The charge has to endure long enough to ensure that the battery is stable.

What we know of sleep comes from studying our brainwaves (with an electroencephalograh, or EEG), and our behavior, as we sleep. Normal sleep includes the sleeper moving from wakefulness through stages of lighter sleep to deeper sleep stages associated with delta frequencies, also referred to as slow wave sleep. The cycle repeats throughout the night.

1. Stage 1, or non-REM 1 (non-rapid eye movement 1), is shallow and we are half-awake and half-asleep. Non-REM 1 is only supposed to comprise 2% to 5% of our sleep. An increase in this stage is a sign of sleep disturbance.
2. Our sleep gradually deepens into Stages 2, 3, and 4 non-REM phases. These cycles are 80% of a night's sleep.
3. Then we transition to REM (rapid eye movement) sleep.

After the short REM phase, we cycle back into non-REM stages, and the whole process happens again, with each cycle lasting between 90 and 120 minutes. Most people experience from three to seven such cycles per night. When sleep experts like me advise that you get enough sleep, we want you to pass through all three sleep stages, four to five times each night. A good eight-hour sleep allows you to move through five cycles.

REM sleep is characterized by rapid eye movements, paralysis of most muscles other than the diaphragm, and the presence of dreaming. REM sleep makes up about 20% of our sleep and tends to increase during the second half of the night. The first REM stage is short, maybe 10 minutes, and it becomes longer through each cycle, possibly up to 60 minutes. Dreams generally occur in the REM stage of sleep.

The standard unit of measure for any type and frequency of waves is hertz (Hz), which refers here to the brain wave cycles per second.

Brain Wave Type	Cycles per Second (Hz)	Focus	Sleep Cycle	Quality of Sleep
Beta	13–30	Focus on external world	Transition to sleep Mostly beta waves; moves quickly to theta (about 5 min)	
Alpha	8–12	Relaxed wakefulness with closed eyes	Light sleep (shortest cycle)	Relaxed muscles Body does not act out Can have swirling colors and lights Muscle twitches and jerks, loss of sensory awareness
Theta	4–7	Light sleep Mostly dreamless Creative ideas	About 50% of the sleep cycle Waves of slower pace and larger amplitude Sleep spindles, at a higher	Harder to awaken and doing so, you could feel drowsy, foggy, or confused when coming

(continued)

(continued)

Brain Wave Type	Cycles per Second (Hz)	Focus	Sleep Cycle	Quality of Sleep
			frequency, and K-complex waves with greater amplitude occur	out of this sleep Most likely time for sleepwalking to occur
Delta	0–3	Slow wave sleep Deep sleep, little conscious recall	Deep sleep composed of 20% or more delta waves with slow waves and higher amplitude	Supports immune system health Release of human growth hormone Heart and muscle activity slow down for repair and renewal Blood vessels dilate to provide cell nourishment Raises melatonin Reduces levels of the stress hormone cortisol
Brainwave activity returns or cycles through theta and then through beta	4–8 through 12–38	Dreaming sleep supports long-term memory repair and brain health	REM sleep with dreaming	REM sleep occurs at the end of each sleep cycle

Understanding the sleep stages and cycles can help you plan when to go to sleep and when to awaken for maximum benefit. For example, if you tend to go bed at 11:00 p.m., read a book, and drift off to sleep about 11:30 p.m., your ideal waking time might be after four sleep cycles, which would bring you to 7:30 a.m. If you felt you needed more sleep, you would go to bed at 10:00 p.m. to allow completion of five sleep cycles. Four cycles of undisturbed sleep may render you fresher and feeling better in the morning than your friend's sleep of five cycles in which her cat disturbed her sleep on and off. Experiment to find out what works best for you.

The Effect of Too Little Sleep on Your Health

For the majority of people who get inadequate sleep, the human brain and body experience alarming symptoms. The research is conclusive:

1. The National Sleep Foundation estimates that over 30% of the population sleep less than six hours at night. What is the big deal, you ask? Sleep is a critical cornerstone of good health. Sleep is the opportunity for the body to restore balance. When that doesn't happen, internal systems break down over time.
2. There is a direct relationship between the lack of sleep and the obesity epidemic. Insufficient sleep causes an increase in the release of *ghrelin*, an appetite-enhancing hormone secreted by the stomach that makes you want to eat. At the same time, it causes a decrease in the secretion of *leptin*, an appetite-suppressing hormone produced by fat cells. This, in addition to the fatigue caused by insufficient sleep, leads to weight gain. Unfortunately, this is a major problem in children as well, and is a contributing factor to childhood obesity.

3. Insufficient sleep also causes insulin resistance, which can contribute to a diagnosis of type 2 diabetes. The American Diabetes Association is now publicizing the fact that adequate sleep is an important part of treating diabetes.
4. Inadequate sleep also results in cognitive dysfunction and sleepiness. If you have insufficient sleep, you tend to underperform at work. You have difficulty concentrating, focusing, remembering, and you tend to become easily irritated.
5. Breaking new research has found that lack of sleep and poor quality sleep can compromise your immune system and inhibit your immunological reaction to infection. In one study, people deprived of sleep for a few days following an influenza vaccine had a much lower immune response as measured by antibody production when tested two weeks after vaccination.

Abnormalities in your immune system's responses to fighting infections or diseases sometimes create inflammatory conditions such as allergies, asthma, heartburn, or ulcers. Chronic inflammation moves beyond the local organ or tissue, where it starts as a healing agent, and moves into the blood vessels and organs. When this happens, the changing characteristics of inflammation are now "systemic inflammation."

In one sleep study, researchers tested and examined the participants' specific levels of three inflammatory markers. These three markers are associated with a higher risk of atherosclerosis, predisposing one to heart attacks and strokes:

1. Fibrinogen (blood-clotting protein)
2. Interleukin-6 (proinflammatory and anti-inflammatory cytokine)
3. C-reactive protein (CRP levels in blood rise in response to inflammation)

Participants with poor quality sleep had higher levels in all three inflammatory markers while those who slept six to nine hours had lower levels. The conclusion of the study indicated:

1. Poor sleep quality and short sleep durations are associated with higher levels of inflammation.
2. Normalizing sleep quality and duration reduces the risk of inflammation in cardiovascular disease.
3. There is a direct link between lack of sleep and hypertension and cardiovascular disease. If you are chronically sleep deprived, your body produces excessive amounts of the stress hormones adrenaline and noradrenalin. The result is progressive blood pressure elevations. Additionally, when you sleep, your average blood pressure drops by 10 to 15 points. Sleeping less deprives you of several hours of this important decrease in blood pressure that you should be experiencing every night. According to Professor Francesco Cappuccio of the University of Warwick Medical School: "If you sleep less than six hours per night and have disturbed sleep, you stand a 48% greater chance of developing or dying from heart disease and a 15% greater chance of developing or dying of a stroke."
4. Lack of sleep can exacerbate multiple sclerosis. A recent study revealed that cells that produce myelin, the nerve-insulating material that is destroyed in multiple sclerosis, double in production during REM sleep and are destroyed in sleep-deprived mice. (Because mice and humans share the brain's ancient circuitry, these findings are important to note.)
5. There is a potential connection to Alzheimer's disease. Another recent study of mice showed that during sleep the process through which cerebrospinal fluid cleanses

the brain of harmful wastes such as beta amyloid, the protein affecting memory loss in Alzheimer's disease, increases tenfold. Lack of sleep compromises this process.

I cannot emphasize enough how an uninterrupted night of solid eight-hour sleep can help maintain good health and improve both emotional stability and mental functions.

Fatigue and Brain Fog

Sandy appeared more than just tired during our consultation. The word *exhausted* came to mind, as I quickly scanned the dark circles under her puffy eyes. Her shoulders sagged as if she were holding the weight of the world. I welcomed her and asked, "How can I help you today? Are you not sleeping?" My bit of humor in asking if she had come to a sleep clinic because she wasn't sleeping well flew right over her head.

Rather, Sandy focused mentally on her story, and with scrunched brows, she began: "I am not sure I've slept well now for the past year—about the time my husband of 30 years needed emergency heart surgery. We got through that, and he gained back the weight he lost before the heart surgery. His snoring also returned because he now sleeps on his back. I seem to spend the night waking him up to ask that he turn on his side, and then I can't sleep at all."

"Sandy, were you sleeping better before his heart surgery? Were your patterns of sleep different?"

"Hmm, well, thinking back, every time he gained a lot of weight, he snored more. So I woke up several times a night, and I tossed and turned a lot. I could tell when I was tired because I'd take a nap, pass out, and just be dead to the world . . . maybe about once a week. Now and then he tried to wake me up to make sure I wasn't dead."

I laughed at her humor, but she did not. She was dead serious. My mind started clicking through my mental file of symptoms, checking for types of insomnia, possible patterns of sleep deprivation, and reviewing her sleep hygiene. I asked, "Sandy, did your husband come with you today?"

"No."

"Any particular reason why?"

"I didn't want him to come. I want to find a way for me to sleep first, and then I can help him with any sleep issues. I read your sleep column in the paper on sleep apnea, and I think he might have that. But . . ."

I waited. She seemed to forget what she was saying. "Sandy, you were saying you wanted to see me first. Why is that?"

"Yeah. I did, and forgetting like that in the middle of conversation is one reason. I am forgetful. My brain is mush most of the day, although I seem to do okay at work. Sometimes I run home on my lunch break and just take a short nap. A power nap, I think it was called in a magazine. Even 10 minutes helps."

"Does a power nap really help?"

"Truthfully, no, in regard to sleep, in that I can rest for 10 minutes and stare at the wall, but I am not asleep. Then I don't want to go back to my secretarial chair for five more hours."

I asked Sandy further questions about her sleep routines and behaviors. In the process, she hinted at the fact that she had shared a bed with her husband all the years of her marriage. She asked if sleeping alone would help her.

"I am not sure, Sandy. We won't know how you might sleep until you give it a try, and I can help you with that. You can create a quiet, dark sleeping space, and that will be a good start. Is that one reason you came to the sleep clinic?" She nodded, and Sandy and I concluded her sleep history.

After her appointment, Sandy thanked me and said she might try sleeping by herself for a while and see if she felt any better. She made a return appointment for herself and one for her husband also.

Sandy was true to her word and brought her husband to the sleep clinic. Casually, she told me that she had moved to a cooler, downstairs bedroom to sleep. Her fatigued appearance had improved.

I saw most of the symptoms of sleep deprivation in Sandy: sleepiness (nap at noon), fatigue, problems with attention and memory, and cognitive impairment (brain fog) in that she couldn't make a firm decision about changing sleeping arrangements, Months passed before she could decide to get help, and her mind ruminated on such issues in those hours of lost sleep. I also documented that she woke up often during the night to ask her husband to change sleeping positions. I suspect she did not reach the restorative sleep stages.

In summary, Sandy's sleep disturbances and the resulting symptoms fed each other and created a vicious circle:

1. *The environment:* Her sleeping in the same bed, and even the same room, with a bed partner whose sleep apnea and weight contributed to her lack of sleep.
2. *The lack of deep sleep:* Sandy awakened consistently throughout the night, keeping her from the deeper, restorative stages of sleep.

The results of sleep disturbance? An increase in stress hormones, high blood pressure, and all the signs of emotional agitation, mental fatigue, and daytime sleepiness.

I feel it's important to note that Sandy was only 48 years old. You may have thought she was older based on her many years of marriage, her husband's sleep apnea and heart disease, her fatigue, and her slowness at work. Many of her symptoms are typically associated with aging. But sleep disorders are happening at younger ages. You could meet a Sandy who is 18 or 28 years old. Sleep rejuvenates, and those who do not create the space and goal of coveting it for themselves will sound just like Sandy.

Take the First Step and the Rest Falls into Place

What can you do to improve your sleep?

First, come to the realization that you need at least seven to nine hours of sleep each night. Not accepting this one fact could have profound costs for you, including your suffering from diabetes, heart disease, stroke, or obesity—all of which link to a lack of sleep.

Second, practice good sleep hygiene as outlined in the next chapter to get those hours. This may involve changing long-held habits and modifying your behavior, but I hope the information in this chapter will motivate you. Good sleep brings clear thinking and vitality. I encourage you to value sleep and allow yourself to embrace a lifestyle change to improve your entire outlook and health. Instead of thinking of sleep as a necessary evil, think of it as a valued commodity you invest in. Instead of thinking of sleep as a recurring event that robs you of valuable time, think of it as a luxurious opportunity to find peace. Sleep is transformative. If you value your life and want to enjoy better health, then deep sleep is your prized ally.

3

How to Get a Good Night's Sleep

For you to sleep well at night, the aesthetic, the quality, has to be carried all the way through.

—STEVE JOBS

What motivates you to get up each morning and enjoy your day?

No matter what it is, whatever motivates you to get up each morning will also motivate you to change poor sleep hygiene and adapt to better sleep habits.

Identify Your Motivation

Adaptation means to adjust by learning new behaviors that allow you to cope with change. At first, adaptation seems hard, especially if you are like Sandy and too tired to take action, and too mentally fatigued to care or to research your options, all because of disrupted sleep. Sandy also had sleep habits and beliefs that kept her stuck in poor sleep. Sandy could have moved into a separate bedroom long before she came to see me, but I felt she needed permission to do so. She felt guilty even *wanting* to sleep alone.

Take a few moments now and use these three steps to identify your own motivation and develop better adaptation skills:

1. Make a list of what you know to be happening, not what you *think* is happening. Sandy's list included going to bed at the same time each night, listening to her husband snore, waking him up, feeling unable to get up in the morning, having coffee and going to work, feeling limp by 10:30 a.m. . . . you get the idea. Sandy thought she was helping her husband, when the reality was she was hurting herself by continuing the same sleep pattern night after night. When she looked hard at her list, the light bulb went on, and she was motivated to change her sleeping habits.

2. Ask yourself what is the worst thing that could happen if things don't change. Sandy's worst fear was that if she died, her husband would be alone, with no one to care for him. Facing that fear was more motivation for her to make changes right away.

3. Adopt a purposeful approach to changing poor sleep habits or making new habits a part of your life. Change one habit at a time and then give yourself the time to make it real and good for you. How much time do you think Sandy needed to move to a separate bedroom? After talking with her husband, one evening was all the time it took. However, Sandy then woke up throughout the night listening for him. That habit took about 10 days to pass. Even though Sandy had five habits to change on her list, by acting right away on the first two, the other three disappeared and she threw the list away.

Create an Ideal Bedroom Environment

Your bedroom environment plays a critical role in your ability to sleep well. Simple changes can yield quick results. Design and organize your own sleeping space as a sanctuary where you can retreat from the stress of everyday life and sleep well every night.

Lighting: Cover windows with dark curtains, shutters, or fabric so that no light shines in.

Bright light wakes you up! Exposure to dim light at night affects your moods, possibly pushing you to depression. Exposure to blue lights emitted from electronic devices is beneficial during the day in stimulating your attention, moods, and even your reaction times. Take an electronic device to bed, however, and it keeps you awake. Of all light-wave frequencies, red light is the least disturbing to moods and to sleep. Plug-in nightlights with red bulbs are available.

Room temperature: The cooler the room, within limits of comfort, the more likely you are to fall asleep. One of the major signals that occur with the onset of sleep is a drop in core body temperature. If your room is too warm, this drop is inhibited, making entering sleep more difficult. I suggest a room temperature of around 68 degrees because this harmonizes with the drop in your body temperature about four to five hours into sleep. The Sleep Foundation discourages temperatures above 75 degrees Fahrenheit and below 54 degrees Fahrenheit, as they will disrupt sleep. If you are having trouble falling asleep, try regulating the room temperature.

Sound: You need your bedroom to not only be cool and dark, but also quiet. If a dripping faucet or the barking of a neighbor's dog is interfering with your sleep, try earplugs, earphones, or generating white or pink noise to even the sound field so your ears won't focus on the background contrast of environmental sounds. There are machines available to do so, but for some the sound of a fan will do the trick. If your partner's snoring is keeping you awake, you should encourage him or her to be checked by a doctor for sleep apnea. Treatment can improve your sleep and also might save his or her life.

Alarm clock: Watching an alarm clock is another problem when you cannot fall or remain asleep. It causes two sleep-opposing reactions. The first reaction is calculating time, which results in speeding up of your brain waves and making a return to sleep very difficult. The second reaction is provoking anxiety due to mental rumination about *how much sleep will I get* or *how will I function tomorrow*. This causes the release of stress hormones such as cortisol, which normally are at their lowest levels during sleep. The rumination then makes it difficult to return to sleep and impossible for the body to reduce the stress hormones and restore some balance. Place your alarm clock somewhere you cannot see it, like across the room with the face to the wall.

Pets: Do not sleep with pets unless they contribute to your well-being. Do not compromise your health because of what you feel your cat or dog may want, need, or demand. Sleeping without them may be a difficult habit to break for all of you; but remember, you're making the change for them as much as for yourself. You will be a much better caretaker and companion if you're healthy and energized.

Design: The hotel chain Travelodge conducted a survey of 2,000 guests as to how room color affects sleeping. According to participants, the best color for sleeping was pale blue. Here are more results:

1. Pale blue in the bedroom was associated with calmness. Fifty-eight percent of those surveyed said they regularly

woke up happy. On average, they reported sleeping 7 hours and 52 minutes.

2. Certain shades of pale yellow were the next color identified by the people surveyed, who said they slept for 7 hours and 40 minutes on average per night.

3. Green (which shade is unknown) was chosen as the third best color for sleeping, and those surveyed reported getting an average of 7 hours and 30 minutes of sleep per night, with 22% of those surveyed saying they woke up "feeling upbeat and positive."

In addition to painting your room in a calm, soothing color, here are more suggestions for making your bedroom a place for renewal and rest:

- Place the bed in the center of a wall, allowing enough room for a chair or nightstand.
- Clear clutter. Stuff shoes or slippers slightly under the edge at the end of the bed, place books on a nightstand (not on the floor), and put away all clothing and children's toys so your room is clear of anything you might trip over in the middle of the night.
- Fill your bedroom walls and ceiling with images, photos, stencils, or painted artwork that help you relax. Here are some ideas of what others have done:
  - One man painted the wall opposite his bed with a lush forest theme, complete with a path meandering through the tall trees.
  - One woman asked her friend, a nature photographer, to blow up images of beautiful flower gardens from his extensive collection. She was delighted to see her small bedroom so full of bright colors. She said, "I smile every time I see the array of colorful flowers."
  - In her young daughter's bedroom, a mom left one wall to paint a different scene each year on her

daughter's birthday. When younger, the scenes included jungle animals, and the next year the same animals were depicted in a circus scene. At age six, her daughter now loves dolphins, and the wall has become a colorful rendition of beach sand, blue sky, and dolphins swimming.

No Blue Lights at Night

Specific cells in the eyes that are sensitive to blue light also regulate your sense of night and day and the seasons. The eyes detect and associate the blue light with daylight. The blue light travels via cells to the hypothalamus, which then shuts down the production of melatonin, one of the major sleep-promoting hormones. If your body does not produce melatonin for sleep and the blue light stimulates you, you are in for a very long night.

Electronic devices: I have had countless patients who cannot fall asleep for hours. However, they are watching their televisions in bed. They are on their computers, playing their video games. Do you do this? Perhaps you do not realize that the blue light from your electronic device is stimulating you to stay awake. Your bedroom should be a sanctuary for sleep and intimacy; eliminate the electronic devices from the room.

Light bulbs: White low-energy fluorescent and LED bulbs typically produce much more blue light than conventional white incandescent bulbs.

Break Habits That Hinder Sleep

Late night nicotine such as the bedtime cigarette is also counterproductive. Many of my patients who cannot fall asleep or stay asleep tell me a cigarette helps them to relax. Indeed, with the first puff this may be true. Nevertheless, within a short time nicotine promotes the release of the brain neurotransmitter acetylcholine. This is one of the most powerful wake-promoting chemicals produced by our brain. It increases the activity of the major wake-promoting circuit of the brain called the reticular activating system.

Alcohol is another problem. It initially can induce sleep and can promote increased deep sleep. Unfortunately, many fall into the drinking trap, because as your body metabolizes alcohol, this causes a withdrawal characterized by an increase in the release of stress hormones such as adrenaline and noradrenaline. This then results in a rebound of wakefulness, causing an inability to return to sleep.

Caffeine-containing foods such as coffee, caffeinated teas, and dark chocolate should be avoided if you have trouble sleeping. I usually recommend to my patients with insomnia that they eliminate all caffeine. If they cannot comply with that request, then at least curtail caffeine intake after 10:00 a.m. Some patients have severe headaches and anxiety when they stop cold turkey. For these patients, I recommend a 50% reduction every two days until they are off caffeine.

Habits to Aid Sleep

Taking a warm bath before bedtime can help to induce sleep. A warm bath will raise your body temperature. Exposure to room air after exiting the bath cools you down. A drop in body temperature is a potent signal to the body to enter sleep.

Morning sunlight is the cheapest and most widely available sleep aid. Exposure to sunlight within two hours of awakening is a strong signal to your circadian clock. It helps you to synchronize with your environment and promotes a normal sleep time the following night. That is why sleeping late on the weekends and exposing yourself to light late in the afternoon can desynchronize your internal clock and lead to problems getting up for work on Monday.

Shift workers working the night shift are a special case. They often have problems reorienting their inner clocks to a completely new and, for many, unnatural sleep–wake schedule. If you are a shift worker, I recommend bright light at work, especially during the first half of the shift. This promotes wakefulness and alertness. However, on the way home when the rest of us are just getting up, you need to get ready to fall asleep. To facilitate this, I suggest that you wear sunglasses that wrap around to prevent sunlight from hitting your retinas. In fact, there now are glasses that specifically screen out blue light. This part of the light spectrum is the most potent in facilitating wakefulness, and yes, I speak of the same blue light emitted by your electrical devices.

Dismiss a Worry or Dump an Attitude

Check worries at the bedroom door. Too many people take their worries into the bedroom, which makes falling asleep very difficult.

Scott was a delivery driver for an international beer company in his small territory located in an area of the Colorado Rocky Mountains. He started driving his truck as a young man fresh off the ranch and a new high school graduate. He was excellent in his work because he greeted hundreds of people a week, and tens of thousands every year, and remembered every name and face. He developed a powerful physique from loading and unloading those crates of beer for 20 years. Everyone admired him.

One day, Scott didn't appear for work, and his manager called numerous times and finally went to his home. His boss found Scott on the floor and guessed he had a heart attack. Scott was very lucky to recover and returned to work, but not before having a serious talk with his manager, who thought Scott was going to quit. The manager would offer whatever incentive he could to keep his valued friend and employee.

"Scott," said the manager, I need you to stay on with the company and take over my job as manager. I just don't know anyone who can befriend and care for people like you do."

"I don't want the job."

"What? But when I offered it to you last month, you said you would think about it."

"I did think about it . . . sitting in your chair day in and day out . . . missing my friends and customers along the routes. Heck, Jim, even my big Shepherd dog knows everybody like I do. Sitting on this tile floor all day would kill him, too."

"Are you saying you don't want the raise or promotion?"

"I guess that is what I'm saying. I went to bed each night of the last 29 days, and I'd worry so long and hard, that I'd sweat and toss and turn. After a couple weeks, I just yelled into the night, 'What am I afraid of?' Next thing I know, you found me on the floor, boss. I don't remember getting up."

"What worried you so much, Scott, that it gave you a heart attack?"

"Heck, that's easy . . . not driving . . . not seeing my customers . . . not stopping by the diner to have my bacon and tomato sandwich with Jules . . . not keeping my great abs."

"Okay Scott, you like what you do, and people love you. Why change a great job? I'll tell you what, Scott . . . I am giving you the raise anyway, and please stick with me."

Scott's story speaks to a good-hearted young man who was lucky to love his work, and his work loved him, despite its physical requirements. He was a people person, and supplied his people with great emotional connections for years. His heart condition was caused by prolonged stress and lack of quality sleep. Scott's anxiety was acute and exacerbated by no sleep or poor quality sleep. Returning to the job he loved was his best medicine. Acute distress and anxiety can happen to anyone, and the following two techniques, constructive worrying and the brain dump, can help you fend off or alleviate any escalating stress symptoms.

Constructive worrying: In the evening, make a list of your problems or worries. Place the list in a drawer and leave it there. No need to act on them. Getting the worries out of your mind and onto the sheet of paper, where you can see and acknowledge the list, is enough to calm the mind.

Brain dump: Have you ever attended a workshop or seminar where the facilitator passed around a wastebasket, going from person to person, and asking for your brain dump? You lower your head over the trash can and shake out all thoughts and become clear and focused for the meeting or seminar. Sounds silly, doesn't it? Yet, it works. Try it before sleeping if worries turn through your mind like a merry-go-round.

Superb Sleep through Progressive Muscle Relaxation

Edmund Jacobson, MD, once said, "An anxious mind cannot relax in a tensed body." Dr. Jacobson studied the relationship between tension and the varied results in health disorders. He developed a progressive muscle relaxation technique to relieve tension in the body. Based on this technique, I've created the following relaxation sequence for my patients. You will feel the benefits right away.

The goal of progressive muscle relaxation is to relax your mind and body by alternating between tensing and relaxing muscle groups. In this exercise, you will tense and relax muscle groups without straining. As you tense each group, take a slow breath through your nose and exhale through your mouth. Even better, inhale while tensing the muscle group and exhale as you relax the group. Try to tense each group for 5 seconds and release and relax each group for 10 seconds.

The total experience is to relax and feel the rhythm . . . tensing, relaxing . . . inhale and tense, exhale and relax. Remember to keep breathing as described above throughout the exercise.

Find a comfortable and quiet place to lie down, such as a couch, bed, or mat when practicing. When you feel you are adept at doing this, move the exercise to the bedroom. Focus on the muscle group you are working. Focus on the breath. If your attention wanders, return to the breath and that muscle group.

1. Begin by progressively tensing the muscles in your feet by curling your toes for a count of 5 as you breathe in, then release the tension as you breathe out and pause for a count of 10.
2. Repeat the process with your calves, thighs, and then buttocks.
3. Now tighten the muscles of your abdomen. Do this by inhaling again, holding for a count of 5, and then relaxing for a count of 10.
4. Then do your lower back by gently arching it for a count of 5, release, and relax for a count of 10. Remember to keep taking those nice gentle breaths and feel the tension released from the muscle as you exhale.
5. Proceed to your hands by making fists, then flex your biceps, and then tighten your triceps by extending your arms out and locking your elbows. Breathe out and pause for a count of 10.
6. Next, inhale and tense your shoulders by lifting them as if to touch your ears, remembering to hold for 5, then release, and relax for 10.
7. Tighten your chest by taking a deep breath in, hold for a count of 5, and exhale, releasing all the tension.

8. Work on your neck by gently pulling your head back, as if you were looking at the ceiling, and continue the breathing pattern.
9. Next, go to the muscles of your face and smile widely, feeling your mouth and cheeks tense and then relax. Work on your forehead by lifting your eyebrows as high as you can.
10. Next, relax your eye muscles by tightly shutting your eyes for a count of 5, exhale, and relax for 10.

You may want to do this exercise in this order, or you may find a different progression works better for you. You could do both extremities simultaneously, or one side at a time.

Finally, feel free to vary the breathing counts as it suits your breathing and comfort. The more you use this specific exercise, the more you will come to appreciate its valuable benefit to help you relax and fall asleep or return to sleep.

What's Next?

If you've tried these best practices to achieve longer, restoring sleep and are still having trouble falling or staying asleep, start keeping track of how you sleep by keeping a sleep diary for at least two weeks. I've provided a sample at the end of this chapter.

Your sleep diary is like a mirror reflecting your sleep–wake cycle. If you have noticed that you are more irritated, tired, and frustrated, or that you cry easily, can't concentrate, or have blank memory moments, then a sleep diary will be your best friend. The diary provides the answers to your inner detective that searches for clues to your unrest or discomfort. In your sleep diary, you or your partner can record sleep quality, waking time, quality of focus and energy during the day, and naptime and quality of rest.

If you have a restless mind, also record the thoughts that keep you awake. Finally, you'll write the time of going to sleep and the time of any night awakenings. After two weeks of recording your pattern, you'll clearly see your sleep–wake cycle map and understand why you feel as you do each day.

A sleep expert will want to review this information. Although self-reporting may not be the most reliable, it does tell your health professional what is important to you, how you view the situation, and enables him or her to discern deeper patterns or issues to address.

As you move to the next step and read the chapters associated with the symptoms you identified on the Sleep Disorder Checklist and implement strategies suggested in them, I hope you will see positive changes in your sleep pattern. However, if your symptoms persist for more than three days a week for over a month, it is time that you spoke to your health care professional. Your sleep diary will provide essential information for a diagnosis.

Sleep Diary

Please fill out sections A and B for each day.

Name:_____ **DOB:**_____

Starting Date:_____ **End:**_____

Date:_____

A. Answer in the Morning After Waking for the Day

	What time did you first go to bed last night?	Approximately how long did it take you to fall asleep?	About how many times, if any, did you awaken during the night?	Overall, about how many hours did you sleep?	What time did you wake up (for the last time) this morning?	In general, how did you feel when you woke up?
DAY 1						o Very refreshed o Somewhat refreshed o Fatigued
DAY 2						o Very refreshed o Somewhat refreshed o Fatigued
DAY 3						o Very refreshed o Somewhat refreshed o Fatigued
DAY 4						o Very refreshed o Somewhat refreshed o Fatigued
DAY 5						o Very refreshed o Somewhat refreshed o Fatigued
DAY 6						o Very refreshed o Somewhat refreshed o Fatigued
DAY 7						o Very refreshed o Somewhat refreshed o Fatigued

B. Answer at Bedtime Just Before You Go to Sleep

	How much time, if any, did you spend napping during the day?	Did you consume any of these substances during the day?	On a scale of 1 to 5, how would you rate your overall mood and overall functioning during the day?
DAY 1		o Caffeine (within 6 hr of bedtime) o Alcohol (within 1 hr of bedtime) o Medication (type:_____)	o 5 – Positive and energetic o 4 o 3 o 2 o 1 – Depressed and lethargic
DAY 2		o Caffeine (within 6 hr of bedtime) o Alcohol (within 1 hr of bedtime) o Medication (type:_____)	o 5 – Positive and energetic o 4 o 3 o 2 o 1 – Depressed and lethargic
DAY 3		o Caffeine (within 6 hr of bedtime) o Alcohol (within 1 hr of bedtime) o Medication (type:_____)	o 5 – Positive and energetic o 4 o 3 o 2 o 1 – Depressed and lethargic
DAY 4		o Caffeine (within 6 hr of bedtime) o Alcohol (within 1 hr of bedtime) o Medication (type:_____)	o 5 – Positive and energetic o 4 o 3 o 2 o 1 – Depressed and lethargic

(continued)

B. Answer at Bedtime Just Before You Go to Sleep (continued)

	How much time, if any, did you spend napping during the day?	Did you consume any of these substances during the day?	On a scale of 1 to 5, how would you rate your overall mood and overall functioning during the day?
DAY 5		o Caffeine (within 6 hr of bedtime) o Alcohol (within 1 hr of bedtime) o Medication (type:_____)	o 5 – Positive & energetic o 4 o 3 o 2 o 1 – Depressed & lethargic
DAY 6		o Caffeine (within 6 hr of bedtime) o Alcohol (within 1 hr of bedtime) o Medication (type:_____)	o 5 – Positive & energetic o 4 o 3 o 2 o 1 – Depressed & lethargic
DAY 7		o Caffeine (within 6 hr of bedtime) o Alcohol (within 1 hr of bedtime) o Medication (type:_____)	o 5 – Positive & energetic o 4 o 3 o 2 o 1 – Depressed & lethargic

PART TWO

Impaired Sleep or Dyssomnias

This category of sleep disorders refers to issues in getting to sleep, staying asleep, and the excessive sleepiness caused by disruptions of sleep duration, quality, or timing of sleep. There are 30 sleeping disorders in this category; here, I've addressed the five most prevalent: restless legs syndrome (RLS), periodic limb movement syndrome, insomnia, circadian rhythm disorder, and sleep apnea.

4

Restless Legs Syndrome

The amount of sleep required by the average person is five minutes more.

—WILSON MEANER

Joan arrived at the Sleep Disorders Center, casually dressed in jeans, and appeared comfortable as she sat down in my office. I noted in her medical history that she was 45 years old. She carried a journal with her, opened it, and stuck her thumb in between the pages to hold her place during our preliminary small talk.

"Hello, Joan, and welcome. It looks like you have some information to share."

"I do. Do you want me to dive in and present my case, or do you want to ask me questions?" Since Joan was ready to read her journal to me, I asked her to proceed.

Joan shared her notes. "About eight weeks ago, I woke up around 2:00 a.m. to this intense tingling in my legs. The longer I stayed in bed, the sensation of tingling became like something crawling slowly up my legs. Of course, nothing was there. I tried propping pillows under my knees and changing positions, but I just had to get up. I could only compare the growing sensations of pain to thousands of pin-pricks. This is hard to describe, so you can see why I wrote it all down. I got out of bed, slid down the wall to the bath-room, and ran some hot water. All I could think of was soak-ing those sensations away. That pattern subsided around 8:00 a.m. I've had two more episodes in the past eight weeks, and I did my homework. I think I have restless legs syn-drome, and I wondered what you would prescribe for that."

"Well, Joan, before I prescribe anything, if I do at all, I need to get a few more facts from you. Can we do that now?" She nodded yes.

"First, Joan, I am going to read nine phrases and you can say yes or no if this sounds like what you experienced, okay?"

"Go for it!"

1. *"It just makes me want to move."*
   "Definitely."
2. *"It feels like I have water running underneath my skin."*
   "Nope."
3. *"It feels painful."*
   "Incredibly so."
4. *"It burns and aches."*
   "Sometimes the tingling could feel like burning, but not aching per se."
5. *"It feels like I have a toothache in my leg."*
   "Don't know what that means. I have never had a toothache."
6. *"I have the heebie jeebies in my legs."*
   "Oh my gosh. I have never heard anyone use that phrase but my father. He said he got the heebie jeebies. He said he had trouble sleeping all the time. You don't suppose his heebie jeebies were leg pains do you?"

Joan seemed excited by the possible connection. I said, "I don't know, but I will be taking a brief family history. RLS sometimes has a hereditary factor. If this is the first time you've had this event, then likely it is not hereditary. Most children in families with a genetic factor have RLS in their childhood, and surely by age 20. So, shall we finish?"

7. *"My legs feel creepy, crawly, and tingly."*
   "Yes."

8. *"It feels like I have worms or bugs crawling deep in my muscles."*
   "Yes."

9. *"It feels like electricity in my legs."*
   "The tingles could be like that a little. Can you diagnose me yet?"

I laughed and gave Joan credit for her persistence and for doing her homework. I appreciate patients who read and search for answers, and even when they think they have an answer, I still have to conduct the history and examination. When patients like Joan experience strange sensations that wake them up and grow in intensity through the night, they fear it happening again. Somehow being able to put a name or diagnosis to a symptom implies that a doctor will be able to provide a solution.

"Joan," I explained, "I still want to conduct a neurological exam. I will review your medical records for medications and such. We have more to do before I can offer a final diagnosis. If that works for you, let's move to the next step."

"Whatever it takes, doctor, you lead the way."

"Basically, Joan, to meet the diagnostic criteria, you would need to have:

1. Symptoms that are severe at night and usually subside during the day.
2. The irresistible urge to move the legs or arms because of pain, burning, pricking, tingling, or numbness.

3. The sensations following relaxation or a period of staying still, and during sleep.
4. Relief from these sensations during movement."

Joan's diagnosis did turn out to be RLS, and further medical tests revealed an iron deficiency. These tests included checking her serum iron for the amount of iron in the blood; her serum ferritin for the level of iron stores her body had used; and her transferrin, the protein that carries iron in the blood, to determine the level of transferrin that was not carrying iron. The first step in treatment was for Joan to rebuild her iron stores, and the RLS was eventually eliminated.

What Is Restless Legs Syndrome (RLS)?

There are two types of RLS:

Primary RLS has no known cause, and stands alone, not being associated with any other disorder.

Secondary RLS can be caused or is associated with a number of disorders including iron deficiency, renal disease, diabetes, multiple sclerosis, and Parkinson's disease. Other known contributors of RLS include alcohol use, muscle overexertion, prolonged sitting, dehydration, and certain medications, such as antipsychotics, antidepressants (except Wellbutrin), and antihistamines (such as doxylamine often used in over-the-counter sleep aids and diphenhydramine (Benadryl)).

RLS is "one of the most prevalent neurological disorders in Europe and North America, affecting about 10% of the population, with women being afflicted almost twice as often as men." Twenty percent of women have RLS symptoms during their third trimester of pregnancy. RLS is often common in people with fibromyalgia. In fact, one-third of women with fibromyalgia have RLS. This is believed to be attributable to the fact that both may be related to abnormalities of the dopamine system. Surveys have demonstrated that 25% of the adults with RLS trace the onset of their symptoms to between the ages of 10 and 20. RLS is a significant contributor to both depression and anxiety disorders, probably due to sleep disruption.

Although commonly overlooked in children, about 2% of American children experience RLS. Unfortunately, past cases of children with RLS were misdiagnosed as "growing pains" and more recently as attention deficit hyperactivity disorder (ADHD). Inattention and hyperactivity among children are associated with symptoms of RLS and may actually be a manifestation of RLS. Further evidence from the survey of clinical studies (up through 2005) confirmed the association between ADHD, ADHD symptoms, and RLS. If your child has been diagnosed with ADHD, consider ruling out RLS or another sleep disorder to ensure the most effective treatment. (For more on ADHD and sleep disorders, see chapter 13.)

There is a strong genetic component. The genetic tendency in those suffering from RLS is a 40% chance of having a first-degree relative with the disease. In fact, the incidence is more than 90% in identical twins. A red flag for inheriting the disorder is the onset of symptoms in early life. One study to determine the age of onset in 250 adults with RLS found a distinction of onset between patients with family histories and those without the family etiology. The peak of onset occurred at 20 years of age, and a smaller peak of onset at 40 years for those with a familial component. Early onset is associated with increased severity, higher incidence of periodic limbs movements in sleep, and movements with micro-arousals during sleep resulting in a disrupted sleep pattern.

No one knows the exact cause of RLS, though a dopamine imbalance in the brain is highly suspected due to a decrease in dopamine levels in cerebral spinal fluid. Dopamine is a neurotransmitter that sends chemicals for muscle control.

Symptoms

1. The characteristics of RLS are the strong urge to move, accompanied or caused by uncomfortable or distressing skin sensations of the legs.
2. People with RLS have unpleasant sensations in the legs, but the sensations can extend into the torso and arms.
3. Patients have described the sensations as
   a. An itch you can't scratch,
   b. Aching muscles, penetrating pain,
   c. An unpleasant tickle that won't stop,
   d. Phantom limb pain,
   e. Crawling, as you brush the crawling thing off your arm, except when you look, nothing is there.

The unpleasant part of these sensations is they can start when you are watching television, reading a book, trying to sleep, or in that space of being awake, yet relaxed. Then the itch, cramp, tickle, or throbbing intensifies into discomfort that is usually relieved by movement like getting out of bed or the chair, walking slowly, and standing, then increasing the movement and stretching if possible.

These sensations tend to occur in the late evening and during the night. The solution is to walk for relief, or even trying Joan's method of a soak in hot water to relax.

Treatment Options

I believe RLS is a disorder of the central nervous system, revolving around the metabolism of the neurotransmitter dopamine. More people with low total-body iron stores, measured by a blood test called ferritin, have a high incidence of RLS. Iron is necessary for the formation of dopamine and explains why the most successful medications in treating RLS stimulate brain areas receptive to dopamine action. On a positive note, iron therapy normalizes ferritin levels and can resolve the disorder in many patients.

Treatment of RLS takes into consideration how to relieve symptoms, but also any discovered cause or associated medical condition such as neuropathy. For relief of RLS that seems sporadic, movement, stretching, and massaging the legs does help to relieve symptoms. You can also make life-style changes such as:

● Eliminating caffeine, nicotine, alcohol, and over-the-counter drugs containing doxylamine (such as NyQuil) or diphenhydramine (Benadryl), since all of these sub-stances seem to aggravate RLS.
● Moderate daily exercise such as a 20-minute power walk or yoga stretches.

If symptoms persist, ask your health care provider to test you for low levels of iron, magnesium, and potassium. If necessary, you may need to add supplements to your diet. Other effective treatments not involving medications are pneumatic compression, massage, near-infrared light therapy, and programs of physical activity. Pneumatic compression involves a compression garment "sleeve," also used to prevent blood clots from forming after surgery, that fits on the arm or the leg. Attached to the sleeve is an electric pneumatic pump that fills the garment with compressed air on a timed cycle. The cycled compression helps lymph to pump and blood to circulate.

In other studies in patients with spider veins, varicose veins, and other superficial varicosities, both sclerother-apy, in which a medicine is injected into the blood vessels to make them shrink, and laser ablation have proven to be very effective. In a recent study of laser therapy, there was an 80% success rate.

The Difference between RLS and Periodic Limb Movements

A common misconception is to label involuntary movements of the limbs during sleep as RLS. These are periodic limb movements in sleep, and cause insomnia and daytime sleepiness. Although they are more common in people with RLS, they are not the same disorder. The differences are listed here.

Periodic Limb Movements	Restless Legs Syndrome
Are involuntary	While the syndrome can occur when one is asleep or awake, the patient can voluntarily respond and act on the pain
Are nocturnal	Can occur rarely during day and are primarily nocturnal
Patient not aware of the movement	Patient is aware
Movements occur repetitively	Sensations or pains in RLS are mostly continuous sensations that grow in intensity

Answers to Your Questions

Over the years, I have received numerous questions about RLS. RLS is a significant contributor to both depression and anxiety. I hope that my answers to these questions will help you:

1. Understand how people experience the varied symptoms of RLS.

2. Become more aware of the medications available for RLS, and know their side effects.
3. Pay attention to the onset of unusual symptoms and discuss them with your doctor.

FOOT PAIN AT NIGHT

Q. My husband has a problem with his feet. They hurt him so badly that at night he cannot stand to have anything touching them. He sleeps with the bedcovers off. His feet even go numb occasionally. He was tested for diabetes, but that was negative. Can you think of a reason his feet would hurt like this?

A. The question is, do your husband's feet hurt only at night and when immobile? If this is the case, it might be RLS. On the other hand, if this is an ongoing problem regardless of the timing, and moving his legs does not relieve symptoms, this could be neuropathy. Although diabetes is a common cause of neuropathy, there are numerous other causes. Have a neurologist evaluate your husband. Many tests can determine the cause.

RLS AND ANTIDEPRESSANTS

Q. I consulted with a psychopharmacologist. I mentioned that I had RLS. He told me that the antidepressants like the one I was taking could cause RLS. Since stopping the medication, I no longer have an irresistible urge to move and rub my legs. I thought you might want to pass this on to your readers.

A. Thank you for your suggestion to address this important issue. It is true that almost all antidepressant medications can cause or increase the symptoms of RLS. There is, however, one exception, and that is bupropion, also known as Wellbutrin. That is why I frequently recommend

Wellbutrin as the antidepressant of choice for a patient with RLS.

WHY DO I RUB MY FEET TOGETHER?

Q. To get to sleep I must rub my feet together. I simply cannot sleep unless I do that. Sometimes this may go on for up to an hour before I can fall asleep. What is wrong with me?

A. What you are describing could be RLS. People with RLS tend to develop their symptoms after dark. They frequently experience an irresistible urge to move or rub their legs. This is a common cause of an inability to either fall or stay asleep.

ARE GAMBLING AND RLS RELATED?

Q. I have heard that there is a link between RLS and a gambling addiction. Do you know anything about that?

A. Yes, I do. However, the RLS itself is not associated with compulsive gambling. It is one of the medications used to treat RLS. There is a risk that the medications for RLS could exacerbate problems if you struggle with compulsive shopping, gambling, or binge eating. Please note that this is a very rare occurrence.

RELATIONSHIP BETWEEN RLS AND OBSESSION

Q. My wife has RLS. She started on a medication called Requip. Since starting on it, she goes shopping every day, and it is costing us a lot of money. Is there any relationship? It seems like too much of a coincidence.

A. Requip and some of the other medications used to treat RLS such as Mirapex have been associated with impulse control disorders. Problems include compulsive gambling, shopping, or eating, and hypersexuality. These problems were reported in up to 7% of those using these medications. I would definitely bring this to the attention of your health care provider.

A NEW MEDICATION AND LEG TINGLING

Q. I have severe acid reflux. Four months ago, my doctor started me on the medication metoclopramide since the Prilosec I was taking was not effective. The new medication works. However, for the last few weeks, my legs drive me crazy at night. I get some tingling sensations that can only be relieved by walking or rubbing my legs. I think this might be RLS. Could there be a relationship to my new medication?

A. The answer to both questions is yes. What you are describing is a classic example of RLS. Although it is not definite, the metoclopramide is a likely cause. Metoclopramide (Reglan) blocks the activity of a brain chemical called dopamine. This blocking effect on dopamine may be the basis for the development of RLS. It is important that you point out the symptoms to your physician.

RLS PAIN AFTER NEW MEDICATION

Q. I have had RLS for several years. I have been on a medication called Sinemet all this time and have been fine. Recently, the pain has returned and the symptoms are starting earlier in the day. It is worse than ever and has started in my arms as well. What could be happening and what can I do?

A. What you are describing is, unfortunately, very common with the medication Sinemet, also known as carbidopa-levodopa. The condition is *augmentation* and affects 70% of patients on this medication for RLS. The pain worsens and occurs earlier in the evening and may spread to other parts of the body. I recommend that you see your health care provider. You need to switch to a different medication such as Requip, Mirapex, or gabapentin. Increasing the dose and frequency of Sinemet will only make matters worse.

RLS CORRELATION TO ATTENTION DEFICIT HYPERACTIVITY DISORDER (ADHD)

Q. My brother takes a medication called Ritalin for ADHD. He is 23 years old and can't sit still. Recently, I read that a disorder called RLS is related to ADHD. Can you explain this relationship?

A. At a recent meeting of the American Academy of Neurology, a paper was presented pointing out this relationship. In 40 patients with RLS, 39% had ADHD, while in a controlled group without RLS, less than 15% had ADHD. The authors feel that this leg discomfort can cause people to be hyperactive and distractible. You may be on to something with your brother. Advise him to discuss this with his doctor. There are numerous new medications available to treat this disorder.

RLS AND SLEEP ATTACKS

Q. I have RLS. Recently, I was placed on a medication called Mirapex. Friends have told me that there have been reports of people falling asleep suddenly when on this medication. I drive to work every day. Should I be concerned?

A. What you are referring to is "sleep attacks." The truth is they are very rare. Moreover, they have been noted in people with Parkinson's disease who take doses many times higher than what is used for RLS. As of now, I am unaware of any reports of sleep attacks in patients with RLS.

RLS AND EXERCISE

Q. I have RLS. Is there an exercise program that could help me prevent the discomfort I feel that keeps me from sleeping?

A. Unfortunately, no exercise program cures RLS. However, stretching the legs before bedtime has proven helpful in some patients with RLS.

RLS AND NONPHARMACOLOGICAL TREATMENTS

Q. I have RLS and do not like taking medications. Is there anything I can do that does not include oral medications?

A. Yes. Although not as successful as medication, non-pharmacological treatments are available. These include improving sleep hygiene with a regular sleep–wake time, avoiding caffeine, alcohol, and nicotine and, lastly, performing moderate daily exercise. Some patients report that acupuncture and massage are helpful. These modalities have not yet been scientifically studied.

RLS OR FIBROMYALGIA?

Q. I've had fibromyalgia for 10 years. My legs hurt at night, and I get some relief by rubbing and moving them. I heard at a support group that this was part of my fibro-myalgia. However, I have seen on the Internet that this could be a sign of RLS. What do you think?

A. I think you are correct. We know that RLS is very com-mon in people with fibromyalgia. In fact, in a recent study published in the *Journal of Clinical Sleep Medicine*, RLS was 10 times more common in those with fibromyal-gia. In addition, you state that the symptoms occur pre-dominantly at night. That is a key characteristic of RLS.

I recommend that you discuss this with your primary care provider.

RLS AND VARICOSE VEINS

Q. I have RLS. It keeps me from falling asleep, sometimes for hours. It also bothers me when I am in the car and my legs are not moving. I have varicose veins and my legs swell. I am thinking of seeing a vascular specialist. Will this give me relief?

A. In sclerotherapy, a chemical irritant is injected through the skin to close unwanted varicose veins. Several studies have shown improvement in symptoms of RLS. In one study consisting of 113 patients with RLS and varicose veins, 72% of those treated who had relief were maintained at two years. There are some contraindications to the procedure such as active inflammation in the vein. However, if you have not been able to get relief with commonly used medications or have experienced unwanted side effects, it would appear to be a reasonable alternative.

Self-Check: Restless Legs Syndrome Checklist: URGE

Even though RLS is one of the most common neurological disorders in North America, there's no real test for diagnosis. However, there are four key points that doctors use to diagnose RLS. They can be described using the word URGE.

If you think you may have RLS, and this sounds like what you're experiencing, use this URGE acronym when you talk to your doctor.

U = URGE	Urge to move the legs	Leg movement accompanied by uncomfortable sensations deep in the legs that may be described as tingling, creeping, crawling, itching, or burning
R = REST Induced	Rest periods of inactivity are when the urge to move gets worse	Inactivity like resting, sitting, or lying down is when RLS typically hits
G = GETS better with activity	Movement such as walking or stretching brings relief	Unpleasant sensations reappear when you stop
E = EVENING and night	The urge to move increases in the evening or at night	Or occurs only in the evening or at night

Insomnia

Insomnia is a gross feeder. It will nourish itself on any kind of thinking, including thinking about not thinking.
—CLIFTON FADIMAN

Do you experience difficulty falling or staying asleep? Do you wake often during the night or have restless sleep? Insomnia is the most common sleep disorder in the United States, affecting approximately one of every three people. Insomnia in younger adults typically manifests itself as a difficulty to initiate sleep, whereas in older adults, insomnia tends to cause a difficulty in maintaining sleep. You may have had temporary bouts of insomnia, called transient or acute adjustment insomnia, going through a divorce, losing a job, or losing a family member in death. Fifteen percent of those one-in-three persons with bouts of acute adjustment insomnia eventually go on to suffer from chronic insomnia.

Primary Insomnia

Ally was 21 years old, and a recent education graduate of the state university. Her soft-spoken voice gave way to more enthusiasm and ease as she discussed why she came to the Sleep Disorders Center, "My mom encouraged me to come see you. What she tells me, now that I've been home most of the summer applying for teaching jobs, is that I seem snappy and irritable. Sometimes I talk faster, like I'm brushing off her questions. I will say that this is true because I feel tired. Her house is hot, and I don't sleep well at night as it is. I am trying to adjust living with her again. Then we get into an argument. Sometimes I cry. She says I cry a lot."

Searching for sleep disorder clues, I asked, "Ally, I appreciate that your mom sent you to the Center, as she must feel you don't sleep well. What's your take on how you sleep?"

"Hmmm, I don't think I really sleep but for a few hours here and there. At night it seems I worry a lot, and so I try and keep myself busy. I watch a little television, fill out job applications, or keep up with college friends on Facebook. Mom doesn't like it, but now and then I might have a glass of wine that she reserves for us only at dinner."

"So a few hours here and there means . . ."

"Well, if I go to bed and lie there, sometimes I see a couple of hours have passed when I check the clock in between trying to read a few pages of a book or texting a few friends. You know, that just gets old, so I get up and then find something to do to take my mind off not being able to sleep."

"Good, next are your nighttime rituals new? Or, did you do these night activities before you went to college? And how about when you lived in the dorm?"

"Mom had a cancer scare when I was 12. Yes, in high school, I worried all the time. I heard her squeaky bed every time she turned over, and listened intently to make sure she turned again. Man, I was hyper back then . . . maybe I still am. Then when I was dating, I always made curfew, and still worried about her. The house is so small, and I've never seen Mom smile much at all."

"Ally, let me summarize this for a moment. In high school, your mom had a cancer scare, and that triggered in you this worrying at night, listening for her bed noise to make sure she was okay, or perhaps still alive?"

"Yeah, it's true. I used to shake in bed at night I was so afraid she would die. That was when I was 12, and sometimes I'd stay awake in my room and color, read, do homework, or talk to my girlfriends late at night because I didn't want to cry in bed."

"Ally," I said, "you are very clear in your descriptions, but there is one point that I want you to be certain about. I realize you associate your worrying at night with the trauma you and your mom went through around your early teen years. Yet, people adapt, and you would have let go of the cancer moment in your teen years.

"The fact that the sleep patterns are still going on had to shift into a habit of not being able to fall asleep whether or not you thought about your mom. Can you remember when you realized that you just couldn't fall asleep, and the longer you stayed in bed, the more you worried about falling asleep and all the repercussions that would have on you the next day?"

"Like, how do you mean?"

"I mean that from age 12 forward, what started as worry and fear around your mom and cancer has grown into an anxiety about going to sleep. The bedtime rituals you started and continued through your teen years have become a perpetuating habit that keeps you from sleeping, as hard as you try. Can you remember a shift in your worry patterns from the subject of mom to the subject of going to bed?"

Ally felt her anxiety turned from her mom into not being able to fall asleep or wanting to go to bed somewhere between her junior and senior years. She shared that she would take a book to bed, and read . . . waiting to be sleepy. Rather, she tended to be more awake. She would watch the clock, turn over, read some more, and finally get up.

In college, Ally learned to drink alcohol with friends, and she felt this helped her sleep better, but she still woke up within one to two hours after going to bed, and rarely returned to sleep. During all-night study sessions, her friends took amphetamines, but she drank caffeine–colas or coffee all night. In college, she scheduled her courses so she was always in her dorm room in the afternoon to "study and sleep." However, she never slept.

Now that she is living with her mom again, she does drink wine, but has reverted to the same bedtime rituals, and subsequent anxiety about sleep.

Ally's story reveals how a smart teen developed insomnia over time as fears and worrisome thoughts took hold within her brain and body. She developed sleep-preventing behaviors and associations that made falling asleep almost impossible without the use of alcohol or medications for sleep. Any symptoms her mom may have noticed were masked in comments like "teens always sleep in, drinking alcohol is just part of college life, the hot bath relaxes me, I am handling *it* . . ."

When a mental health screening ruled out anxiety as a primary disorder, Ally learned her diagnosis was *psychophysiological insomnia*, one of five types of the most common primary insomnias that affect 15% of the population in the Unites States. Primary insomnia patients are moody and anxious, especially around sleep and bedtime. Ally had developed severe anxiety and muscle tension associated around her inability to fall asleep and the bedroom environment. Over her teen and college years, she developed hyperarousal, a state of being constantly alert at night, and developed rituals at night that served:

1. To delude Ally into thinking she was taking care of herself.
2. As sleep-preventing behaviors, which created poor sleep habits.

Another way to understand the development and continuance of primary insomnia is through the three-Ps, which are predispositions, precipitating factors, and then perpetuating variables or conditions.

Predispositions	Predisposing factors include genetic, physical, or psychological patterns that make certain persons hyperresponsive or more susceptible. For a deeper understanding of those characteristics in persons' nervous systems that make them overly responsive, I refer you to Elaine Aron's popular book, *The Highly Sensitive Person*.
Precipitating	These are events or influences that push a person into patterns of acute sleep disruptions.
Perpetuating	What perpetuates insomnia are behaviors implemented to relieve insomnia, but end up making the insomnia worse, or conditions that prevent establishing normal sleep. *Behaviors*—like staying in bed and trying to sleep, which exacerbates not sleeping. *Psychological*—like continuing to worry about an issue. *Environmental*—like sleeping with lights on or with a loudly snoring bed partner that keeps you awake. *Physical factors*—like a chronic illness or pain.

Our goal was to help Ally start again with sleep habits and rituals that supported her health. We began with sleep hygiene, stimulus control, and a cognitive behavioral therapy (CBT) technique called cognitive restructuring.

SLEEP HYGIENE

Ally was instructed to eliminate all caffeine including chocolate within 12 hours of bedtime. She was to refrain from looking at the alarm clock at night and put it in a place where she could hear it but not see it. Following the protocol, Ally removed the television from her bedroom, refrained from using any electronic devices within two hours of bedtime, and no longer did her work in bed at night. In fact, we wanted her to associate her bedroom with sleep and nothing else.

STIMULUS CONTROL

As part of stimulus control, we instructed her to follow this sequence:

1. Not to nap during the day.
2. Get into bed when truly sleepy.
3. After 20 minutes, if wide awake, leave the bedroom.
4. Go into another quiet room to read or listen to soothing music.
5. Return to bed when she once again felt sleepy.

COGNITIVE RESTRUCTURING

Ally was told to recognize and write down her numerous dysfunctional beliefs about sleep, such as, *"If I don't get enough sleep I'll be miserable. I know this is destroying my health. I must have at least eight hours of sleep to function. All my problems are due to my poor sleep."*

Next, she was to write and rehearse in her mind more positive modifications of these negative thoughts, such as, *"I've been through this before, and I'm able to function. I've had this problem for a while and my health is excellent. I can't blame everything on my sleep. My doctor explained to me that we need five and one-half hours of what is called core sleep to function adequately. We may not feel great but we can function. He explained that most insomnia sufferers underestimate the time that they are actually asleep."*

It took a few months but she kept at it. We could see in her sleep diaries that she was falling asleep sooner and staying asleep. At first she went from five to six hours total sleep. In the end it was seven and one-half hours and she felt great.

There were minor relapses over the next few years, but she would then reinstitute the techniques she had been taught, and in very little time she would be back to seven to eight hours of quality sleep.

This is why we prefer CBT as opposed to medications for people such as Ally. CBT is a form of psychotherapy or counseling, with varied techniques to help you regulate the way you think, as well as behaviors. CBT is used for persistent insomnia as the primary disorder, as well as with coexisting disorders. CBT is long-lasting because it reverses the actual underlying behaviors, associations, and dysfunctional beliefs. Medications seem to work while being taken, but most people's problems return when medications are stopped. We'll discuss CBT techniques in more detail later in this chapter.

SYMPTOMS

You also may be one of the 30% of the population with insomnia. This sleep disorder includes:

1. Inability to fall asleep.
2. Inability to stay asleep.
3. Early morning awakenings and not feeling renewed or refreshed.
4. Feeling as though your sleep is of poor quality or is nonrestorative.

These sleep patterns affect your ability to function each day. You may wake up tired and be less mentally alert. However, most insomniacs are not sleepy, which is more like feeling drowsy or tired. They are more likely to complain of fatigue, which is not the same thing. They feel as if they have no energy and have to push themselves to get things accomplished. Do you remember a scary night from your childhood in which you laid awake, still, and alert all night? That constant, vigilant state is hyperarousal that places the nervous system on an extremely taxing chronic alert. Imagine holding that tension for days, for weeks, and then for months. How many would be capable of functioning normally? In short, insomniacs hold such tension and thus suffer from frequent and severe fatigue.

Transient Insomnia

Maria was a resilient woman who lost her mother at age 17. She stayed with her best friend and her family, graduated from high school, and hit the streets. After years with the wrong crowd, Maria finally found a good job with a strong, mentoring employer who sent her to college and helped her achieve healing with a therapist through the company's medical program. The street girl went straight, married a policeman, and presently has two children, Jenny, age four, and Matt, age two. She had already experienced the new mother's sleepless syndrome, by the time she came to see me.

"Doctor, I am here because I was diagnosed with a rare form of rheumatoid arthritis last week, and I haven't slept a wink since. I've already been to a nutritionist, understand this will be a life-long disease, and I worry. All night I pretend to talk to my husband while he snores away. Then I talk to my dead mother, and sometimes to God about what will happen to me. What will happen to my children? The pain is supposed to get worse over the years . . . I need help. When I lie awake all night, I cry all day. My husband thinks I am going off the deep end, but I tell him it is just no sleep. No sleep and I cry. Thinking of my kids with no mom, I cry . . . can you help me?"

Maria's case is a classic example of transient, or acute adjustment insomnia. Maria was so anxious over her medical diagnosis that she could not sleep. This had been going on for less than a month so it had not yet become chronic. Maria was smart to come to the Sleep Disorders Center early on in her lack of sleep. She had not yet developed sleep-preventing behaviors such as napping during the day, excessive caffeine intake to stay awake, or clock watching in response to her inability to sleep, to mention just a few of the symptoms that would develop if her insomnia persisted, as Ally's had.

This is one of the situations where I provided a short-term use of an approved sleep medication. I gave Maria an initial two-week prescription for a sleep aid to use only if she was unable to fall asleep after several hours. Research has shown that restorative sleep does improve the physical and mental stressors Maria experienced. I also discussed sleep hygiene and bedtime relaxation techniques. I asked Maria to call me within two days to let me know how it worked for her. I also referred her to a therapist as it was obvious that more than just a sleep aid was necessary to help her cope long term with her diagnosis.

For patients like Maria, early intervention is incredibly important, which is why I let such patients clearly know that a short-term medication is step one of a larger coping process. If Maria continued to go without sleep, it was unlikely that therapy would be of much help. In fact, the acute condition was more likely to develop into chronic insomnia associated with depression, a disorder which is very common in chronic pain disorders and much more difficult to treat.

Insomnia with Multiple Causal Factors

Tom's primary care physician referred him to me for several reasons. Tom, an insurance agent who worked long hours, was overweight and had been waking up in the middle of the night for months. An inability to maintain sleep is a common symptom of insomnia. Tom's doctor wrote in his records that he had been unable to stay asleep for at least four months, had trouble focusing at work, and had great fear of a heart attack because of his lifestyle. Tom's wife had slept in a separate bedroom for some time due to Tom's snoring, so there was no one to observe Tom's awakenings or to verify any of his symptoms.

According to Tom, he woke each morning somewhere around 2:30 to 3:30 a.m. He reported waking up and feeling anxious. His mind would be racing and his thoughts frequently turned to work. In fact, he frequently took out his laptop and reviewed the next day's work. He was a smoker, and if working on the laptop did not ease his anxiousness, he would light up a cigarette, as it seemed to relax him.

After a while, Tom turned off the laptop and the lights to go back to sleep. It rarely worked. In fact, most of the time after waking at 3:00 a.m., Tom stayed awake in bed until 6:00 a.m. when he needed to get ready for work. Those early morning hours for Tom were grueling because of his racing mind.

His sleep habits on the weekend were no different except that he stayed in bed until 8:00 a.m. His anxiety rose in those early morning hours. His daytime mental abilities were foggy and unfocused. He was moody. Finally, Tom was so frustrated by the lack of sleep and the lack of results of his efforts that he dreaded going to the bedroom. He had become so anxious about his inability to fall asleep that now he was having trouble falling asleep. His primary care physician was wise to send Tom to me first because sleeping well could turn his life around, and Tom was desperate to do so.

To determine Tom's problem, I needed to sort through several symptoms. Early morning awakenings had become a chronic problem with negative consequences such as fatigue and irritability. Tom had poor sleep hygiene such as caffeine intake, alcohol use, and staying in bed and doing work-related activities when unable to return to sleep. He also had an insomnia severity score of 27, which was consistent with very severe insomnia, and a General Anxiety Score (GAD-7) of 16, also high, and consistent with his reports of his racing mind. There was no indication of depression from his assessment.

After we'd identified the symptoms, my job was to sort through them and reverse the situation. The process was time-consuming, but the detective work is well worth the end result. Possibilities included a breathing disorder, sleep apnea, or a rapid eye movement (REM) sleep disorder.

To narrow things down, Tom first needed to work on his poor sleep hygiene and learn how he had developed the counterproductive habits. I explained

- How the blue light from his laptop in the middle of the night would put an end to any chance of returning to sleep.
- That the nicotine of his cigarette was a major stimulant promoting wakefulness.
- That he could not make himself return to sleep, and the harder he tried, the more anxious and awake he became.

- That lying in bed not sleeping was far worse than getting out of bed and doing something peaceful and soothing.
- Consistent rising with an alarm every morning would help reset Tom's circadian clock.
- No naps in the afternoon after work would make sleep more likely moving forward.

I explained the behavioral technique called stimulus control, discussed later in this chapter. This treatment focuses on reducing exposure to things that cause wakefulness at night, and the goal is to establish immediate sleep and an optimal sleep–wake cycle. If Tom did not fall asleep within 20 minutes after waking, he got out of bed and chose to stay in the living room area with no computer and read. He avoided stimulating activities, and if he got sleepy again, he returned to bed. If he still could not sleep then he was to return to the living room and do something that was relaxing.

We also used cognitive restructuring, delving into Tom's dysfunctional beliefs about insomnia. Focusing on thoughts like *this lack of sleep will give me a heart attack* only made matters worse. However, Tom could affirm his sleep as restorative and healthy.

Tom went home with several weeks of sleep logs to be filled out in the morning after he was awake and out of bed for the day. He would bring these back for his weekly appointments.

My hope was that these strategies would correct his insomnia. If not, my next step would be a sleep study to determine if sleep apnea was the root cause of the problem. Only recently have we sleep specialists come to appreciate how often an inability to remain asleep or early morning awakenings can be triggered by a primary sleep disorder such as sleep apnea and sometimes by periodic leg movements causing arousals from sleep.

If we still had not resolved the problem, I would consider placing Tom on one of the more sedating anti-anxiety antidepressant medications. I have had great success with these medications when generalized anxiety disorder has been at the root of the problem. The medications are even more effective when combined with CBT.

After a few months there was a significant improvement in that Tom was still awakening in the early morning hours after sleep onset, but he was able to return to sleep in a much shorter time. At this point, bothered by his continued awakening from sleep, I ordered a sleep study. I rarely perform sleep studies for insomnia, but when the insomnia occurs after falling asleep and is persistent despite good patient adherence to therapy, I feel a sleep study is in order.

Lo and behold, Tom did have sleep apnea that was particularly severe at 3:00 a.m. during REM (dream) sleep. This is not unusual, as sleep apnea appears to be more severe during dream sleep in many individuals, and dream sleep tends to increase significantly during the second half of the night. Treating Tom's sleep apnea was an important part of treating his insomnia.

Tom's lifestyle and stressors also contributed to insomnia. Because behavior and insomnia are closely linked, treatment must include the behavior and emotional associations surrounding bedtime and sleeping. Changing sleep practices is one part, and the transformation of feelings and thoughts into more successful habits is the second part.

Chronic Insomnia

In 10% of the population, insomnia is a chronic problem, lasting over three months. In fact, most studies measure the duration of the problem in years.

INDICATIONS

1. Duration of longer than one month.
2. Continuing symptoms on two or more follow-up visits with your health care provider.

Multiple factors contribute to a diagnosis of chronic insomnia, including:

- Heredity in one-third of the cases.
- Mental health disorders such as depression, anxiety, attention deficit hyperactivity disorder (ADHD), post-traumatic stress, or bipolar disorder.
- Substance abuse, the consistent triggering of the hyper-arousal state, and certain medical conditions and medications.

If untreated, many go on to develop depression. In fact, in one study of over 14,000 patients, insomnia preceded depression in 40% of cases. That percentage still amazes me because I see that an insomniac might not clearly recognize his or her personal level of dysfunction. In addition, insomnia occurs at the same time as anxiety disorders in 38% of cases. If you leave insomnia untreated, the relapse rates of depression and anxiety are very high. It also creates high risk factors for other mental health issues, substantial health care costs, dysfunction in work and relationships, as well as decreased quality of life.

A recent study from South Korea, published in the journal *Sleep*, highlights the emotional problems associated with persistent insomnia. In this study, researchers followed over 1,000 people with insomnia for a six-year period. Researchers first eliminated those with insomnia and either depression or suicidal ideation. Over the next six years, researchers closely followed those with chronic insomnia, and screened them periodically for the development of depression or suicidal ideation. The odds of developing depression were 2.5 times more likely and developing suicidal ideation was 1.7 times more likely in those with continuing insomnia. Other published studies that also correlated insomnia with the odds of developing depression or suicidal thoughts were higher than in the Korean study.

If left untreated, chronic insomnia can result in significant emotional consequences. Prevent any transient insomnia from progressing.

Why You Suffer from Insomnia

There are two major schools of thought as to why you might suffer from insomnia. The first is the physiological hyperarousal theory, which means the brain and body stay in an alert, aware state. Insomnia sufferers show faster brain waves that are characteristic of wakefulness and mental processing while asleep. They also produce more stress hormones such as cortisol, adrenaline, and noradrenaline at night. In addition, PET scans show an increase in glucose uptake in the brain while asleep compared to normal sleep patterns.

The second theory is the psychological theory. Insomnia sufferers seem to have anxiety-prone personalities, may be ruminators and worriers, and tend to internalize their emotions. Therefore, they have more trouble dealing with chronic daily stressors such as occupational or family conflicts, as well as major life events such as divorce, death in the family, or illness. For example, insomnia is a risk factor for depression. Recent research on a small sample of people with chronic primary insomnia provided the MRI evidence of the neurobiology "underlying the dysfunctional emotion regulation in people with insomnia" and linked the risk between insomnia and depression.

Obviously, the symptoms of the brain and body coexist and one can exacerbate the other. That is why one treatment does not fit all persons with insomnia. Sleep experts sometimes need to combine pharmacologic treatment with CBT, even if for a short period, to achieve the goal of getting good quality sleep such as in the example of my patient Maria.

Do You Have a Vulnerability to Insomnia?

No matter what your age or gender, insomnia can happen to you. The following is a list of inherent traits and life stressors that could increase your vulnerability to insomnia:

1. Hyperarousal—chronic state of alert.
2. Family history of light or disrupted sleep.
3. Tendency to worry.
4. Anxiety-prone personality.
5. Preoccupation with well-being.
6. Dramatic responses to impactful life events such as surgery, death, birth, loss of job or financial security, illness onset or chronic illness.
7. Environmental factors such as living near traffic noise.
8. How you deal with sleep and insomnia most often perpetuates the insomnia.

Insomnia and Women

Women are two times more likely to report insomnia than are men. Why?

Sleep experts understand that women may have greater awareness of insomnia symptoms. They are more likely to talk about insomnia or mention incidents in social situations and in their roles as mother, caretaker, or wife. While biological differences in a woman's life cycle contribute to insomnia, a family history of a mother's insomnia also likely increases the incidence. Insomnia increases with age, but women's research confirms a steep rise of insomnia in midlife.

The rise is easily understood considering the three phases of menses a woman passes through in the twenty years from age 40 to 60: perimenopause hot flashes, menopause with psychological sensitivity and distress, and postmenopausal possibility of sleep-disordered breathing. Any further factors contributing to persistent insomnia are similar to those in men.

In summary, women are at higher risk of developing insomnia than are men, and treatment considerations must include the stage of the life cycle, predisposition to mood disorders, and hormonal considerations such as nocturnal hot flashes.

Treatment Options

The greatest news is that there are treatments for insomnia that can improve your health, function, and quality of life. The American Academy of Sleep Medicine suggests both pharmaceuticals and behavioral approaches in order to improve sleep.

GOOD SLEEP HYGIENE

Sleep hygiene simply refers to the habits you put in place for better sleep. People can develop counterproductive behaviors referred to as poor sleep hygiene. Constantly looking at the alarm clock, going to bed and staying in bed when not sleepy, attempting to sleep later on weekends or nonwork days, and consuming alcohol to help get to sleep are but a few of these counterproductive behaviors. If you haven't already instituted the suggestions outlined in chapter 3, do so now.

Set a specific schedule of going to bed and waking up. The insomniac's internal circadian clock is out of sync with the sun cycle. To reset your internal clock requires a consistent time for sleep and waking. Your body thrives with a consistent routine. Chapter 6 on circadian sleep disorders explains in detail why the brain and body function best on a set schedule.

STIMULUS CONTROL

With chronic insomnia, you tend to develop negative sleep-preventing behaviors, like severe anxiety surrounding the rituals of going to bed and the bedroom environment. A good night's sleep becomes impossible. In fact, some find it easier to sleep in a foreign environment, such as a hotel or at a friend's house that does not contain stimuli that trigger their anxiety about sleep. I find that some actually sleep better in our sleep lab than at home. Sleep specialists call this Reverse First Night Effects.

This treatment focuses on reducing exposure to things that cause wakefulness at night, and the goal is to establish immediate sleep and an optimal sleep–wake cycle. This therapy helps an insomniac to reprogram negative associations about going to bed, the bedroom rituals, and the environment, into a pleasurable or desirable activity for the specific goal of sleep. Instructions for this therapy include:

1. Go to bed only when sleepy.
2. Get out of bed when unable to sleep.
3. Go to another room and return to bed only when sleep is imminent.
4. Curtail all sleep-incompatible activities.
5. Rise at a regular time every day, regardless of the amount of sleep the night before.
6. Avoid napping.

SLEEP RESTRICTION

This method ensures the time spent in bed corresponds to the actual time you are sleeping, and not the total time spent in bed trying to sleep. You are in bed only to sleep, and you limit the time in your bed not sleeping. You go to bed later but maintain the same wake time, and then increase the time in bed over a specific period, according to your sleep expert's guidance, until you sleep all night.

For instance, you sleep only six hours but spend eight or more in bed. In sleep restriction therapy, the sleep specialist will start you at six and one-half available hours for going to sleep and waking up. The specialist checks your sleep diary weekly to see if you are sleeping more than 85% of the time spent in bed. If yes, then he will extend your total sleep time available in bed by 15 minutes. This sleep time will be extended or shortened weekly, depending on whether you are sleeping more or less than the 85% of time available to sleep.

COGNITIVE BEHAVIORAL THERAPY (CBT)

CBT is a form of psychotherapy or counseling, with varied techniques to help you regulate your thoughts as well as behaviors around sleep. The focus on thinking about how you feel and act helps you become more aware of negative thought patterns that prevent you from changing behaviors. In time, you'll learn how to regulate behaviors using CBT techniques. CBT is used for persistent insomnia, as the primary disorder, along with coexisting disorders.

Cognitive Restructuring

Some insomniacs develop numerous dysfunctional beliefs about sleep. Thoughts listed on page 71 are just a few common examples of what I hear every day from my patients.

Date and Time	Situation	Automatic Thoughts	Emotions	Alternative Response	Outcomes	Notes

- *I know if I don't get eight hours of sleep I'll be miserable all week.*
- *Insomnia is going to severely impact my health.*
- *I just know I won't be able to function.*
- *I'm going to lose my job.*

Is it any wonder that these people cannot get good sleep? In fact, these negative experiences and counterproductive behaviors stimulate the production of stress hormones, making sleepless nights even worse. Cognitive restructuring challenges the person to validate the reality of his or her proclamations.

A sleep specialist may challenge or query in friendly ways: "Let's get a reality check. Show me the evidence for that belief. Let's track your week and see how that thought plays out." The point is to empower the patient to notice and observe, record, write or keep track, and then be accountable to report and process the findings with the sleep expert. CBT is based on the premise that incorrect thoughts lead to emotional suffering and habitual thoughts become embellished. A diary or record of the thoughts and feelings helps you identify and change the habits that do not work for you (see facing page).

Seventy to eighty percent of people with insomnia find CBT provides reliable and prolonged benefits.

ONLINE COGNITIVE BEHAVIORAL THERAPY

This is great for people in locations that do not have sleep specialists and others trained in nonpharmacological treatments of insomnia. These programs are conducted online, and you communicate with someone trained in CBT. You will be offered various nonpharmacological techniques such as stimulus control, sleep restriction therapy, and cognitive restructuring. Your therapist will review your progress weekly and make online recommendations. The treatment period may vary, but the average is eight weeks.

RELEASE TENSION AND RELAX BEFORE GOING TO BED

In my experience, many insomnia sufferers show an inability to close down the day emotionally. They refer to it as being too stressed. In a book called *Sound Sleep, Sound Mind: 7 Keys to Sleeping through the Night*, Barry Krakow, MD, postulates that an inability to identify, feel, and process emotions is what sets many with insomnia apart from good sleepers. The insomniacs think about emotions rather than experience and process them. This leaves them going to bed with their brain on overdrive. Dr. Krakow's theory is that if we learn to feel and process our emotions during the day, we will sleep better at night. Certainly, it would seem to be a better way than medications.

Here are three exercises to help you wind down and release emotional tension at the end of the day:

1. *Noticing*: When a parent notices a child acting out for attention, a common phrase is "I notice that you are . . . paying attention, eating your green beans, picking up your toys. . . ." Noticing the small things is a practice of paying attention, and when you pay attention to your emotions, they dissipate. With your eyes open or closed, feel your way through your body, starting at your head and moving down. Notice if your neck holds a pain, your shoulders are burdened, your expression is tight, your chest feels heavy, or your gut is angered and so forth. When you do notice an emotion, stay with it; or move into the center of it and notice how much lighter the emotion feels.
2. *Noticing with Words*: The "name it and tame it" aspect of emotions includes self-talk. Close your eyes and feel your way through your body, noticing each important emotion as it rises. Then, speak softly the noticing statement: *"I notice my shoulder feels angry. I'm angry at not finishing the conversation with my boss. I accept* [or acknowledge, own, release] *my anger."* Then, you feel your way to the

next emotional area: *"I feel twinges in my gut. The twinge is the emotion disgust. I was disgusted with the way the child in my classroom pushed another, and I did not speak up strongly enough. I acknowledge this emotion."*

3. *Writing What's on Your Mind*: The idea of noticing and accepting our emotions before sleeping is to get the inside out. Writing in a journal may be easier than verbal or visual noticing activities. When you write what is on your mind or in your emotions that bothers you, this form of self-acceptance or acknowledgment in physically writing out the emotions releases any pent-up energy around the issues, as you keep writing long enough to feel the tension dissipate and your breathing become more relaxed.

Any training that helps you relax such as deeper, effective breathing, biofeedback, yoga stretches, guided imagery exercises, and light hypnosis sleep tapes, can be very effective in assisting you to sleep. You choose what you like to do, and would look forward to doing because you would feel better, more relaxed, and quieter inside. These factors motivate you so you don't feel like you "have to" work harder at sleeping or "do one more thing!"

For people with hyperarousal syndrome, several relaxation therapies can help them to retrain this anxiety pattern. I suggest patients undertake this type of intervention with support and guidance, or at least an accountability partner, because a commitment over time is required to establish new patterns in the body. Here are two relaxation approaches:

1. *Progressive Muscle Relaxation.* See chapter 3.
2. *Guided Imagery.* The best way to begin this type of program is to listen to an audio induction that would help you relax while suggesting one imagery set for your focus. The mind is engaged in a pastoral scene, a walk on a mountain trail, or a slow swim through a warm pool.

Generally, these guided scripts last from 10 to 20 minutes, providing the space for the body and brain to relax. Such imagery sequences can also help you sleep better as part of your sleep hygiene changes.

MEDICATIONS

There are several classes of medications available and approved by the FDA for the treatment of insomnia. I do not believe this is necessarily the best approach. However, I think it is important to understand how these medications work.

1. *Over-the-counter sleep aids for insomnia.* Most of these are antihistamines that block histamine, a stimulating wake-promoting neurotransmitter. Undesirable side effects include constipation, urinary retention, dry mouth, and daytime sedation. Most people become tolerant, meaning the drug loses its effectiveness in a short time.
2. *Melatonin supplements* tend to shorten the time to fall asleep and may be effective in certain circadian disorders, such as when you travel and experience jet lag or have delayed sleep difficulties. In addition, melatonin could be effective in the elderly who tend to produce less melatonin. Recent studies have demonstrated its effectiveness in patients on beta blockers. Doctors commonly prescribe these medications for hypertension, heart disease, migraines, and tremors. Beta blockers tend to block the production of melatonin by the pineal gland.
3. *Benzodiazepines* are the medications that target the GABA system (gamma-aminobutyric acid), the most potent sleep-promoting neurotransmitter in the brain. The following medications make this GABA neurotransmitter more potent:
   1. Temazepam (Restoril)
   2. Triazolam (Halcion)
   3. Flurazepam (Dalmane)

4. The newer medications, such as zolpidem (Ambien) and eszopiclone (Lunesta), are *nonbenzodiazepines.* Like benzo-diazepines, they target the GABA system, but they have a different chemical structure.
5. *Medications not developed for sleep, yet commonly used for sleep,* though the FDA has not approved them, include antidepressants such as
   1. Trazodone (Desyrel)
   2. Amitriptyline (Elavil)
   3. Mirtazapine (Remeron)
   4. Antipsychotic medication quetiapine (Seroquel)

Preparing for an Appointment with a Sleep Specialist

If you suffer from chronic insomnia, do not ignore it. Do not wait until you develop a mood disorder. Seek out a sleep expert, who can offer a diagnosis based on your sleep history, medical history, and a possible sleep study if a primary sleep disorder like sleep apnea is considered.

If someone just writes a prescription for a sleep medication without taking the time to discuss your problem in depth, you are probably in the wrong place. Finally, there are prac-titioners skilled in both the pharmacologic and nonpharma-cologic treatment of insomnia in most areas. An excellent resource is the American Academy of Sleep Medicine and the Society of Behavioral Sleep Medicine.

If you decide to see a doctor, pull together the following information:

1. A sleep diary, at least one week's worth (Any patient com-ing to see me with a complaint of insomnia is provided with this at least a week in advance of our appointment.)
2. A list of contributing insomnia factors as you see them
3. A written review of your personal sleep history and habits
4. A summary of how you function during the day

5. A summary of how you cope emotionally and mentally (Are you moody, explosive, withdrawn? Is that emotional coping normal or not normal for you?)
6. A list of what you have tried for sleeping and how you presently manage

Answers to Your Questions

SLEEP MAINTENANCE

Q. I can fall asleep without a problem, but I wake up at least three times per night and cannot fall back to sleep for at least a half-hour each time. Would testing in a sleep lab be helpful?

A. Sleep maintenance insomnia, which is an inability to stay asleep, may warrant a sleep study. What the sleep specialist will be looking for is a possible sleep disorder such as sleep apnea or periodic limb movement that may be causing you to wake up.

CHRONIC INSOMNIA

Q. I have been having trouble falling and staying asleep for about four months. It does not happen every night, but about three to four times a week. Would this be considered insomnia?

A. Yes, it's consistent with chronic insomnia. Chronic insomnia is difficulty falling asleep or staying asleep, as well as early morning awakenings at least three times per week and for greater than three months.

PARADOXICAL SLEEP

Q. My husband returned from Afghanistan last year. He swears he sleeps no more than two hours a night. However, whenever I am awake, he seems to be asleep. I am sure he is sleeping much longer.

A. Paradoxical sleep is very common in returning veterans. In fact, in one recent study, it comprised 15% of all insomnias in vets. In the general population, it is less than 5%. Even though they are asleep, they do not perceive that they are sleeping, in part due to the hypervigilance and alertness they had to maintain day and night while they were on assignment.

DRINKING COFFEE

Q. My wife can drink coffee right up until bedtime and have no trouble falling asleep. If I consume anything with caffeine after 4:00 p.m., I have a hard time falling and staying asleep.

A. Recent studies have shown that those who are sensitive to caffeine may have an inherited predisposition to its sleep-preventing properties. In some people, caffeine consumption disrupts the secretion of the sleep-promoting hormone melatonin, while in others it has little to no effect.

SLEEP DEPRIVATION

Q. My husband sleeps only five hours a night. He claims it is all he needs. However, on the weekends he sleeps at least 12 to 13 hours. We do not have the family time I would like to see him spend with our children. What do you think?

A. Your husband is showing signs of chronic sleep deprivation. One of the major clues as to whether you are getting enough sleep is the "sleep debt." Your total sleep time per night should not vary much on weekends or vacations. The fact that he is sleeping so long on the weekends indicates insufficient sleeping on the weekdays.

STRESS AND SLEEPING

Q. My wife is unable to sleep more than five hours a night. She claims the problem is stress. We are both retired and pretty much have the same routine. Why is it that I have no trouble sleeping and she does?

A. One explanation that stands out is a breakdown of coping skills. In a recent study in the journal *Psychosomatic Medicine*, people with insomnia were compared to a group that slept well. The frequency of minor stressors in their lives was not different between the two groups. However, the group with insomnia perceived their lives as more stressful and relied on "emotion-focused coping strategies." The insomnia patients tended to focus on the underlying negative emotions and took this to bed with them. This resulted in increased anxiety and disturbed sleep. Actual stress events can be the same with you, but how you perceive and deal with it is the difference. Counseling and behavioral therapy may be beneficial to those who suffer with insomnia.

SMOKING

Q. My wife sleeps only a few hours each night. She smokes right up until bedtime and then again when she wakes up. I keep telling her that the smoking is not helping her sleep. Her answer is, "It relaxes me." What do you think?

A. Nicotine initially causes relaxation in some. However, within a short period of time it binds to areas of the brain that release a chemical called acetylcholine. This is a wake-promoting neurotransmitter and definitely will interfere with sleep. I would tell your wife to taper down her smoking, especially around bedtime. Even better, she should quit altogether.

HUSBAND DENYING INSOMNIA

Q. My husband has severe insomnia. It takes him hours to fall asleep. He refuses to speak to our health care provider about this. His memory does not seem to be as sharp as it once was. I'm wondering if his lack of sleep could be the cause.

A. It is hard to say, but lack of sleep could be a factor. Most insomniacs lack delta sleep or what is often called deep or slow wave sleep. This period of sleep is very important to memory, especially the memorization of facts. Although there may be other causes, your husband's lack of sleep could be playing a part. He really should discuss this with his health care provider.

I'VE TRIED EVERYTHING!

Q. I have had insomnia for 10 years. I average about 5 hours of sleep a night. I have tried and failed to improve with medications, hypnosis, meditation, and various behavioral techniques. Is there anything new out there that is safe and effective?

A. The answer is yes, maybe. There is a new type of medication now being tested. It blocks the actions of the major wake-promoting neurotransmitter in the brain called orexin. Several recently published trials have been very impressive, both as to its effects and as to safety. It has not yet been released and is in the process of undergoing further clinical trials.

NO LUCK WITH SLEEP AIDS

Q. I have had trouble sleeping for many years. I get only five hours of sleep out of the eight I spend in bed. I have tried several over-the-counter sleep aids without success. Do you have any ideas?

A. Yes, first you are spending too much time in bed. The more time you spend in bed trying to make yourself fall asleep, the less likely you are going to fall asleep. A behavioral technique called Sleep Restriction Therapy may work for you. Maintain your same wake time but decrease your time in bed to five and one-half hours for the first week. No napping during the day.

Monitor your time asleep versus your time in bed. After a week, if it exceeds 85%, go to bed 15 minutes earlier. If not, do not change your sleep time. Every week that you sleep on average 85% or more of the time in bed you can advance your sleep time by 15 minutes. This is one of the most successful behavioral techniques for insomnia.

STOP THE CAFFEINE

Q. My 72-year-old husband has trouble falling asleep. Most nights it takes him hours to get to sleep. He has a couple of cups of strong coffee during the day, but always before noon. Our health care provider is advising him to stop consuming coffee completely. I read somewhere that caffeine is metabolized in four to six hours, so how will giving up coffee help?

A. Actually, those studies were done on younger people with the majority being under 30. Studies that are more recent have shown that in the elderly population it may take 16 to 20 hours to metabolize caffeine. Therefore, I agree with your health care provider. Eliminating the caffeine for a while to see what effect it has on your husband's sleep seems to be reasonable.

VALIUM

Q. I acquired a Valium from my friend for one night when over-the-counter sleep inducers weren't helping. I took half of the pill and it helped me go to sleep better than Unisom ever has, and with fewer side effects such as palpitations. How can I talk to my primary care physician about this?

A. Valium is a very poor choice as a sleep aid. First, the FDA does not approve it for sleep and it has a very long duration of action—as much as 40 hours. If you are chronically in need of a sleep aid, you should talk to your primary physician about this. There are excellent nonpharmacological treatments available. However, if you need a prescription medication, there are many with far fewer potential side effects and with FDA approval for sleep.

SINGULAIR

Q. I have allergies and asthma and the past six months have been particularly difficult. My doctor started me on Singulair, which took care of my symptoms and really improved my lung capacity. However, soon after starting it, I began having many dreams at night and ultimately I stopped the drug because the dreams were becoming more intense. Several times, I woke in the early morning in a state of panic. In addition, I noticed a wobbly, unbalanced feeling in my legs during waking hours. I know there are other meds delivered by nasal spray and inhaler that do the same thing that Singulair does. If I try those, would I experience the same side effects? I will be seeing my doctor again soon to discuss this and to also inquire about starting the Allergy Easy drops.

A. It is highly unlikely that you will have the same side effects. Singulair (montelukast) has been associated, although rarely, with nightmares and insomnia. It is in a class of medications called leukotriene inhibitors. Most other medications for allergy and asthma are not in this class, and have not been associated with this side effect.

Insomnia problem	None	Mild	Moderate	Severe	Very Severe
1. Difficulty falling asleep	0	1	2	3	4
2. Difficulty staying asleep	0	1	2	3	4
3. Problem waking up too early	0	1	2	3	4
4. How SATISFIED/DISSATISFIED are you with your CURRENT sleep pattern?	Very satisfied	Satisfied	Moderately satisfied	Dissatisfied	Very dissatisfied
5. How NOTICEABLE to others do you think your sleep problem is in terms of impairing the quality of your life?	0 Not at all	1 A Little	2 Somewhat	3 Much	4 Very much noticeable
6. How WORRIED/DISTRESSED are you about your current sleep problem?	0 Not at all	1 A Little	2 Somewhat	3 Much	4 Very much worried
7. To what extent do you consider your sleep problem to INTERFERE with your daily functioning (e.g., daytime fatigue, mood, ability to function at work/daily chores, concentration, memory, mood, etc.)? CURRENTLY?	0 Not at all	1 A Little	2 Somewhat	3 Much	4 Very much interfering

Self-Check: Insomnia Severity Index

If you have difficulty going to sleep or staying asleep, take the Insomnia Severity Index (ISI) and determine your sleeping pattern and discover whether your sleep issue is mild, moderate, or severe. The ISI (facing page) has seven questions and each one is scored. Then you add the seven scores to get your total score. Compare your score to the guide located below.

This index provides a rating scale from 0 (no problem) to 4 (very severe) for each sleep problem. For every issue, please rate the severity ONLY for the last two weeks and *circle* the number that best describes your answer.

SCORING AND INTERPRETATION

Add the scores for all seven items
 Questions 1 + 2 + 3 + 4 + 5 + 6 + 7 = _____ your total score

Total score categories:
0–7 = No clinically significant insomnia
8–14 = Subthreshold insomnia
15–21 = Clinical insomnia (moderate severity)
22–28 = Clinical insomnia (severe)

6

Circadian Rhythm Disorders

I LOVE getting up in the morning! I clap my hands and say, 'THIS is going to be a great day!'
—DICKY FOX from *JERRY MAGUIRE*

Nearly every creature on earth has an internal "clock" that works in tandem with the planet's rotation around the sun. This inner clock regulates how bees gather honey, and it signals birds to migrate. This biological clock, called circadian biology, is governed by the circadian rhythm, the natural oscillations that occur within the 24-hour cycle and regulates eating, sleeping, and much more, as you will see in this chapter. When this rhythm is disrupted, you may have difficulty with delayed sleep, hormone dysregulation, as well as changes in body temperature and moodiness.

Circadian is derived from the Latin *circa* meaning *about* + *dies*, meaning *day*. The primary circadian rhythm within the brain modulates body temperature, muscle tone, heart rate, and hormones' secretions. Yet did you know that the heart and other major organs also have "clocks" which pace the metabolic functions? No wonder that sleep deprivation and sleep disruptions wreak havoc across the spectrum of one's health.

Circadian Biology and a Normal Circadian Clock

Through the systematic study of sleep biology and the observation of sleep behaviors, circadian biology and the genes that regulate the biological processes every 24 hours were discovered. The enormous value in this science is that it provides the framework we now use for sleeping: the sleep stages, how the brain and body work in each cycle, what happens when sleep cycles are disrupted, and how the "right" kind of sleep restores health. I have great respect for this entire evolutionary process of our circadian biology, and I will be the first to tell you flatly that most people totally disregard how delicate and sensitive this circadian biology can be. Some of this disregard is a lack of knowledge, and in other cases, the disregard is blatant until a health issue occurs.

The circadian rhythm regulates our cycles of sleeping and waking in alignment with the outside world. Light is the most important stimulus that resets the circadian rhythm. Other stimuli include exercise, noise, meals, and temperature. For example, the presence of bright light signifies that it's time to be awake (and makes falling asleep difficult), whereas darkness encourages sleep and makes it difficult to wake up. A normal circadian rhythm regulates both sleep, as well as body temperatures, based on a 24-hour cycle.

The main control center of circadian biology is the suprachiasmatic nucleus (SCN). The SCN influences sleep directly in the brain through chemical output or indirectly through release of the melatonin hormone via the pineal gland. Two types of genes control the SCN: Period genes and Timeless genes. These genes produce proteins, "Per" and "Tim," respectively. The function of these proteins is to increase the activity of neurons in the SCN, which regulate waking and sleeping.

The SCN also controls the activity level of other areas of the brain and regulates the pineal gland. The pineal gland secretes melatonin, a hormone that increases sleepiness. Melatonin secretions begin two to three hours before bedtime, and when taken as a supplement, it can be used as a sleep aid to advance the internal clock. Melatonin affects the receptors in the SCN. When the SCN is damaged, for example, an irregularity in the Per gene can result in body rhythms that are no longer synchronized to light and dark. This, in turn, leads to a circadian rhythm sleep disorder.

Any number of biological and lifestyle factors can disrupt the circadian biology. The two main ones include:

Shift work: Starting in the 1960s, people began working in shifts. Industry prophets of the time predicted increasingly more shift work as global industrialization was the "future."

Technology: The technology revolution changed our waking and sleeping rhythms over the last two decades. Thus, we function within a false sense of time that does not match our genetically coded natural rhythm. Our false sense of time robs us of quality sleep and can shorten our hours in sleep. Blue light pollution is the major cause of this.

BLUE LIGHT POLLUTION

The cells in the eye called rods and cones use light to build images. Retinal ganglion cells respond to light and dark. These cells communicate with the neurons at the brain's base that sets your daily circadian cycle. Melanopsin is particularly sensitive to blue light, a band of light in the narrow 400 to 480 nanometer range.

When blue light hits the retina, a signal is sent to hypothalamus, and melatonin production is turned off and delayed by several hours. This results in an inability to fall asleep and trouble in waking up, as melatonin levels are inappropriately elevated in the morning. This is easily explained by 95% of Americans polled by the National Sleep Foundation who reported using some type of electronics a few nights a week within the hour before bed.

So where is this blue light? First, all of your communication devices (cell phones, computers of all types, televisions) emit blue light. Then include the new government mandated compact fluorescent lighting (CFL) and light-emitting diode (LED) bulbs, which give out much more blue light than the old incandescent light bulbs. Is it any wonder that we are seeing an epidemic of sleep deprivation?

As a result, we see the impact of lack of sleep everywhere, in the form of stress, cognitive dysfunction, chronic diseases, mood disorders, and obesity. In fact, in a recent study, hamsters exposed to blue light at night developed cellular changes in an area of the brain called the hippocampus. This part of the brain is very much involved in memory and emotional processing.

So, short of going back to pre-industrial conditions, what can we do to decrease our exposure to blue light and get our circadian sleep–wake cycle back to normal? My suggestions include:

1. Turning off communication devices two hours before bedtime.
2. Using red nightlights in our bedrooms for illumination. Of all light wavelengths, red light has the least effect on melatonin production.
3. Wearing blue blocker sunglasses at night. These are very effective in screening out blue light. I have instituted this strategy successfully with many of my patients.

Blue blocker sunglasses block blue light, which is the most potent wavelength of light in inhibiting melatonin production. Blue light keeps you awake. This product is excellent for shift workers trying to avoid sunlight on the way home. It also works for people with delayed sleep-phase syndrome in achieving the equivalent of darkness at night. Finally, for those who cannot fall asleep because of late-night use of computers, televisions, and all electronic gadgets you love, blue blocker sunglasses allow you to enjoy the devices without causing a harmful circadian shift.

4. Finally, a software app called f.lux that alters the color of your computer display according to the time of day can be found here: justgetflux.com

We are being bombarded with blue light. More than 200 million computers are purchased worldwide per year. We need to be aware of blue light pollution and take measures to prevent overexposure at the wrong time of day to prevent disruption of our circadian rhythm and improve our health.

Circadian Rhythm Disorders

There are six circadian rhythm disorders. If left untreated, the disorders cause a host of physical and psychological problems and disrupt our personal and professional lives. Jet lag and shift work disorders are caused by external factors that result in being out of sync with the normal dark–light cycle. They are also the most common of the circadian disorders.

JET LAG DISORDER

Most of us are familiar with the term *jet lag*; perhaps we've even experienced it while on a vacation or business trip to another time zone. Jet lag is a temporary condition, lasting a few days to a few weeks, usually one day per time zone until our bodies adjust to the new time zone. If the time difference is only an hour or two, there is not much chance of jet lag. A change of three hours or more, however, is often enough to throw us out of sync with the light–dark cycle and cause a disruption of our circadian rhythm. For people who travel for a living, such as pilots, this disorder can negatively impact health, mood, and quality of life.

Jet lag symptoms vary depending on the individual, how many time zones they've crossed, and even the direction in which they've traveled. Studies show that east-to-west travel, where you gain hours, is easier to recover from than west-to-east travel. Most people with jet lag experience a disruption of their sleep—they either have trouble falling asleep if they have travelled east; or they wake too early if they've travelled west. They might also have trouble staying asleep. Other symptoms include trouble concentrating, headaches and irritability, and even problems with digestion and elimination.

For short trips, doctors recommend that the person adhere to their normal or "home" sleep schedule as much as possible. For longer trips, the treatment centers around getting the person acclimated to the new dark–light cycle as quickly as possible, and could include light therapy and melatonin. There is also evidence to suggest that timing meals and exercise can help recalibrate the system.

Symptoms Checklist
1. Disturbed sleep—such as insomnia, early waking, or excessive sleepiness
2. Daytime fatigue
3. Difficulty concentrating or functioning at your usual level
4. Dehydration
5. Stomach problems, constipation or diarrhea
6. A general feeling of not being well

7. Muscle soreness

8. Menstrual symptoms in women

Getting Help

Jerry works for a financial company. Each month, Jerry flies to England for five to seven days. Every other month, he makes an additional trip to France. Even though he's made these trips for almost a year, he still has not adjusted to what he calls his "screwed-up sleep." Jet lag is due to the body clock not adjusting, and sleep difficulties are one of the main symptoms. Dehydration is also a main symptom.

First of all, Jerry can't fall asleep because while it may be 10:00 p.m. in France, it is only 1:00 p.m. in California. He is up half of the night. Then when he has to get up for meetings, he has indigestion. He delivers his presentations in a half-groggy state, even yawning about halfway through his talks. When Jerry returns to the United States and tries to get back into the swing of things in California, the readjustment is stressful, as he cannot concentrate well at the morning business meetings. His manager finds him to be tired and slower in initiating the next month's projects.

How long does it take to recover from jet lag? The average is one day for each time zone. So if he has crossed five to seven time zones, Jerry's body clock will not adjust during a seven-day trip.

Jerry's manager suggested he see me. "Hi Jerry, I understand your manager referred you because your travels are keeping you down?"

"That's a nice way to put it. I feel like I can't sleep and I can't wake up completely. So how do I deal with this jet lag thing, Doc? I've been reading up on the topic, and everybody's got a different opinion."

"Jerry, there is a protocol to follow that I'll suggest, and it has to be followed pretty closely. Let me talk you through it first, and I'll give you the instructions to take with you. The point is to prepare your body rhythm to change to the rhythm of your destination several days before your trip.

1. Prior to leaving on your trip, go to bed one hour earlier each day for three days.
2. Next, if you can get a flight that will bring you to your destination in the evening hours, that's a good thing. If you can't, if people are sleeping in France when you're on the airplane, then you try to sleep.
3. When you arrive, if you do arrive early in the day, don't take any long naps. That will kill you. If you're absolutely exhausted, and you have to take a nap, then try to keep it to 30 minutes or so. That won't cut into your sleep that night.
4. Don't drink any caffeine or alcohol on the plane. They dehydrate you as well as affect your body clock.
5. When you land, obviously avoid caffeine and alcohol if you're trying to get to sleep.
6. Try taking melatonin, as little as one milligram, an hour before bedtime at your destination for the first three days.
7. Finally, get up the next morning and expose yourself to bright sunlight in the morning to try to get in sync."

Jerry seemed very willing to jump into this routine, and remembered one question, "Doc, what about eating? I feel bloated, and have digestive issues."

"Try to eat your meals on the day of travel and on the plane within similar time frames of when people are eating in England or France, or wherever you are going. Jerry, there are obvious benefits to adjusting as best you can, which requires that you know the zeitgebers that adjust the body clock to its normal state."

"Hold on, Doc. What's a zietgeber?"

"Glad you asked that! Zeitgeber refers to the environmental cues that synchronize your body clock to the 24-hour cycle of light and dark."

Jerry nodded and said, "Okay I get it. Sunrise . . . sunset. If I arrive 9 hours later in Paris when my body clock is ready for breakfast at 8:00 a.m. in California, then I have a light dinner and want to sleep, in keeping with the time zone I'm in. But I can't. The zeitgeber of sunlight is gone in Paris."

"Yes, and that is a good thing because you don't want to be exposing yourself to bright sunlight since you'll be going to sleep. If you were to arrive in the afternoon, which means the sunlight hits your eyes, you're going to have more trouble falling asleep at an earlier hour, which is already your problem when you travel east. In that case, wear the blue blocker sunglasses, to avoid bright sunlight in the late afternoon, if possible.

"Then when you wake up the following morning, you should expose yourself to bright sunlight to help you get in phase with your new destination more easily."

"So, if I follow all of these instructions, Doc, how long is it going to take me to get in sync?"

"My goal is that if you have a five-day trip, you should be able to enjoy it without the extreme fatigue. To do that, let me suggest one more point. I want you to start taking a small dose of melatonin at home for two days before your trip. One or two milligrams at about the time you would be going to bed in London or Paris affects your circadian clock without making you groggy. Just a small dose to duplicate what nighttime will be in England. You will re-sync your clock to your destination clock. If you do these things, I would say that instead of six or seven miserable days, your body will adjust within a day or two of landing."

Jerry did follow these guidelines and returned the next month for his appointment. His smile said it all. "You know, Doc, in Paris, I wasn't myself for the first day or so.

After that, I was much better than I've ever been, and by day three, I was feeling great. Thank you, Dr. Rosenberg. I appreciate your help!"

DELAYED SLEEP PHASE SYNDROME

Most of us know people who are "night owls." They stay up very late and are often most productive in the middle of the night. Despite the benign nickname, these people are suffering from a highly disruptive circadian rhythm disorder known as delayed sleep phase syndrome (DSPS).

Unlike jet lag and shift work sleep disorders, DSPS is an organic disruption in the person's internal clock that causes it to run counter to the light–dark cycle of the outside world. People suffering from this disorder cannot fall asleep at a normal time. Instead, they typically turn in between 1:00 and 4:00 a.m.—hence the name "delayed." Their sleep is otherwise uneventful. They typically go to bed around the same time each night, fall asleep easily, and stay asleep for a sufficient number of hours to feel rested.

The difficulty occurs when they try to adhere to a regular daytime schedule. They have trouble getting up for work or school. They report being irritable, tired, and foggy in the morning, with sleepiness decreasing throughout the day. Their mood also lifts as the evening approaches, but then the cycle begins all over again and repeats itself day in and day out.

When people with normal circadian rhythms have been deprived of sleep, they usually go to bed earlier the next night in order to catch up. In those with DSPS, however, this powerful sleep drive is overridden by their "delayed" circadian rhythm. This means they are not able to sleep earlier. After trying to adhere to their school or work schedule all week, they will play catch up with sleep on the weekends, which only perpetuates the disorder. While research is limited, scientists believe people with DSPS may have a longer-than-normal circadian period. Their melatonin and core body temperature fluctuations also appear to be delayed. Some contend that they also are less sensitive to light than others, and the absence of this natural zeitgeber contributes to the disorder.

Symptoms

1. Cannot go to sleep at the time you desire (may appear like an insomnia symptom)
2. Cannot wake up when you want
3. Feel excessively sleepy during the day
4. Inability to wake up at the desired time and excessive daytime sleepiness
5. Depression and behavior problems, due to daytime drowsiness that can lead to academic problems, fatigue, or dependency on caffeine, sleep aids, or alcohol

Getting Help

When Vita came to see me at the Sleep Disorders Center, she explained that she was having trouble in her college coursework because she was not making it to her morning classes on time. Several days a week, she'd turn off her alarm in a sleepy state instead of getting up and going to class.

"I am worried, Doctor Rosenberg, that I've already missed more than I should. The professor has the right to fail me just because I missed so much. The student counselor suggested that I really see a sleep specialist to find out if I could work out a better schedule."

"Vita, what kind of symptoms did the counselor want you to discuss with me?"

"Oh, I wrote them down. I go to bed later than normal people. Now I've heard that all of my life. I go to bed usually between 2:00 a.m. and 3:00 a.m."

"How do you function in your morning classes?"

"I feel groggy all morning, even after a good night's sleep. I attend class, but don't remember much. I have to borrow my friend's recording or read the text to keep up. I am afraid of falling behind, and all my classes over the next three months are morning classes."

"How does the rest of your day go when you wake early and manage to get to class?"

"I feel more alert in the afternoon actually, and after an early dinner, I either study or put in several hours as a typist for a professor's research. Every bit helps you know. Then I hang with friends, study what I missed in the morning. . . . I don't really get tired until the morning hours, and I go to sleep."

"Vita, your computer, television, those new LED bulbs that you say they put in your dormitory room, well they all give off tremendous amounts of blue light. Those lights make it even more difficult for you to go to sleep. Vita, if you can't turn off the computers or your roommates insist on keeping the lights on, you can get yourself blue blocker sunglasses and wear them for about three hours before bedtime. They block out the blue light and help reset your circadian clock. This will help you go to bed earlier. By the way, Vita, don't forget to take them off when you get into bed."

Like jet lag and shift work sleep disorders, delayed sleep-phase disorder can be treated with morning light therapy to wake Vita up, as well as doses of melatonin at night to increase sleepiness.

Vita's designated sleep program was to gradually adjust her schedule to go to bed about 15 minutes earlier per day. Then, when she awakened, she was to get a bright dose of sunlight 15 minutes earlier each day, thus gradually nudging her circadian system until she reached a reasonable sleep–wake schedule.

The second step in Vita's sleep program was for her to take a small dose of melatonin an hour before each night's bedtime. She was to maintain this practice on weekends or she would fall back into old patterns.

Vita did well in her adjustment over time. However, there will be instances when patients like Vita will have difficulty. The solution can be to prescribe a sleep aid or to counsel such patients to adapt their work schedules, if they can, to their circadian disorder. An example would be someone with DSPS getting an evening shift job.

ADVANCED SLEEP PHASE SYNDROME

This disorder is like DSPS in reverse. Those with advanced sleep phase syndrome (ASPS) are known as larks as opposed to night owls. Larks greet the sunrise, are focused and active at dawn and during the ensuing hours, until the lark tires as the day goes on. Typically, they are in bed between 6:00 and 9:00 p.m. and awake far too early—usually around 4:00 or 5:00 a.m. They may feel refreshed, or simply be unable to sleep any longer. Then they experience increasing sleepiness throughout the day. Whereas delayed sleep has negative effects on morning activities such as work and school, those persons with ASPS have difficulty staying awake at night for parties, work, or any social activities. Treatment includes light therapy, typically in the evening, to help advanced sleep phase patients stay up later.

FREE-RUNNING DISORDER

The name of this disorder, free-running, suggests that a person's circadian rhythm is not in sync, or is no longer entrained, with the 24-hour cycle of light and dark. Characteristic of this disorder is a decreased sensitivity to light that keeps one's body clock from resetting its rhythm and regulating sleep. Instead of the normal 24-hour sleep–wake cycle, people suffering from this disorder do not adjust to the light signals or time cues. Their bedtime cycle tends to drift progressively to one hour later to bed and one hour later to wake in the morning. Eventually, their sleep–wake schedule can progress all the way around the clock.

Free-running disorder is most common in the blind, and the primary issues are insomnia and daytime fatigue that impact, to varying degrees, their social and professional lives. About 50% of totally blind people suffer from free-running disorder. Others are able to structure their sleep patterns around cues other than light, such as a routine for their daytime activities.

Of the sighted population, most at risk are adolescent males with onset in the teens through the twenties. It is not as likely to occur after age 30. Free-running disorder is more likely to be secondary to a mental health disorder or evolve from delayed sleep phase disorder.

Such circumstances are so rare that research is qualitative, as in case studies of the patients' situations. For example, I recently read an interesting journal article describing the case study of a 67-year-old man with sight. He carefully recorded every night for 22 years when he went to bed at progressively delayed times, and he did cycle around the 24-hour period about every 30 days. His agoraphobia, a form of anxiety disorder in which the person fears being in public and/or leaving his home, may have aggravated the free-running disorder. Depression accompanied his anxiety.

Treatments for sighted people with this disorder are similar to those for DSPS, including light therapy and melatonin. Melatonin in rather high doses has been effective with blind patients. There is no known cure for this condition, only management, and as of yet, there is no FDA-approved pharmacological treatment.

IRREGULAR SLEEP–WAKE SYNDROME

This circadian rhythm disorder is characterized by an undefined sleep–wake cycle that results in chronic insomnia and excessive sleepiness, or a combination of the two. These sleep patterns have no rhyme or reason and usually consist of sleep for several hours at various times, regardless of whether it is day or night, around the clock; but when you add up these hours, they usually come out to a normal seven to nine hours total per 24-hour cycle. Most of the people with this disorder are elderly and not that physically active, as well as those with neurobiological disorders such as Alzheimer's and people in nursing homes. It is also found in children with intellectual disability.

The goal of treatment is to lengthen the sleep period to a normal length. One of the methods is to teach patients about sleep hygiene, such as keeping the sleep environment cool, dark, and quiet. There are also several supplements and other medications that can be taken to either stay awake or induce sleepiness. Light exposure during the daytime hours is very important; it is also helpful to adhere to a schedule of activities each day. This circadian rhythm disorder is very rare and not well understood, so a combination of treatments unique to the person is required.

Several management tools help those with irregular sleep–wake syndrome reestablish a normal sleep cycle. I encourage people to spend seven to eight hours in bed, with set sleep and wake times. Adhering to a regular schedule is also important, including the use of zeitgebers such as light, meals, and social interactions. Morning and evening treatments of light therapy of 3,000 lux each for two hours (as compared to sunlight that radiates 10,000 lux) has been shown to help establish a normal sleep cycle as well as improve nocturnal sleep in institutionalized patients, and reduce agitation in demented patients.

SHIFT WORK SLEEP DISORDER

I understand what problems shift workers encounter because of my own experiences. When I was a medical resident at Cook County Hospital in Chicago, the medical field had absolutely no knowledge or interest in sleep. We residents routinely worked 30-hour shifts at least once a week in addition to our usual 16-hour days. There were weeks where our work time approached 100 hours. Only recently have training programs come to terms with how dangerous this is, not only for patients, but also for the residents, who can fall asleep while driving home in a very drowsy state. How would you like to be the patient admitted to my service during my 24th hour without sleep?

I can remember some overnight shifts ending at 7:00 a.m. and having just enough time for a three-hour nap before I had to see my 10:00 a.m. patient in clinic. The schedule was grueling and potentially dangerous. I recall rolling down the windows of my little Volkswagen Karmann Ghia in the dead of a Chicago winter in order to stay awake for the drive home.

It was considered a badge of honor to be able to do this. So if a resident complained, our superiors reminded us, "That's how it is and always has been. You just have to tough it out." I should note that most of these archaic practices have been eliminated in the past 10 years as the field of sleep medicine has come to understand the repercussions of shift work and sleep deprivation.

I was once again exposed to this but on a lesser scale when I went into pulmonary and critical care medicine. I'd be on call for my group every fourth week. It was not unusual to get a call at 3:00 a.m. requiring me to come into the ICU and then go straight to my office with little or no sleep.

Shift work, as a sleep disorder, is also the result of external circumstances and can pose risks to health, life enjoyment, and even safety. Most people work the typical nine-to-five day, which is aligned with the natural light–dark cycle and therefore normal circadian rhythms. However, there are many people such as health care providers, police officers, firefighters, factory workers, and truck drivers, who work overnight shifts. This schedule runs counter to the biological signals that tell us when it's time to sleep and time to wake. In order to be diagnosed with this circadian rhythm disorder, the person must "report difficulty falling asleep, staying asleep, or nonrestorative sleep for at least one month, and it must be associated with a work period that occurs during the habitual sleep phase. There are also required effects on impairment of wakefulness."

This shift work disorder has not been given much clinical attention; however, self-assessment surveys show that night workers tend to get less sleep than people who work during the day, usually because of their sleep time conflicting with the daytime activities of their households. For example, a dad who comes home from work at 4:00 a.m. and must get up a few hours later to get his kids ready for school. Those with this disorder complain of insomnia during the day and sleepiness during their work hours, which can lead to impairment. They also have higher incidences of hypertension, obesity, and heart disease. As a result, shift work sleep disorder can result in accidents during work and other activities, such as driving. However, while the data indicates an increase in occupational accidents on the night shift, more research is necessary before a definitive statement can be made.

Treatment and management of this disorder depend on the flexibility of one's schedule. For example, some night workers are able to take a nap before their shift begins, or even during their break while at work. Bright light treatment in the evening hours, combined with limited light exposure in the morning, can help people adjust to their schedule by resetting their circadian rhythm. This disorder is also treated with melatonin, which helps people get more sleep during the day, as well as drugs such as modafinil, to combat excessive sleepiness during their shift. Shaping the pattern of light exposure with combinations of phototherapy and light avoidance (bright light at work, wearing dark glasses on the commute home, sleeping in a darkened room) can shift the circadian pacemaker to a more appropriate phase.

Answers to Your Questions

EFFECT OF LIGHT

Q. Doesn't light affect your circadian rhythm?

A. Yes, light is the strongest stimulus that affects the circadian system. If exposed to light in the morning, one tends to go to bed earlier or at normal time. If exposed to light at night, this will delay sleep.

GETTING UP IN THE MORNING

Q. I recently started a job that requires I be up by 6:00 a.m. I have always had a very hard time getting going in the morning. It can take me over an hour before I feel alert. I'm afraid this is interfering with my job. I'm also concerned about my driving in the morning. Any ideas?

A. Yes. What you are describing is called sleep inertia. Most of us take about 10 minutes to fully awaken. However, some require much more time. Several recent studies have shown that bright light can help. I would suggest that you leave your blinds and drapes open so that you get bright sunlight in the morning. If that fails, there are now clocks that come with dawn light simulators. Exposure to the light has been shown to increase core body temperature. This in turn increases wakefulness.

IRREGULAR SLEEP–WAKE DISORDER AND ALZHEIMER'S

Q. My 78-year-old mother has Alzheimer's and is in a nursing home. She sleeps on and off throughout the day and night. There is no rhyme or reason as to when she falls asleep or is awake. Is this common in Alzheimer's? Is there anything that can be done to help? Most of the time when we come to visit she is asleep.

A. Good question. What you are describing is called irregular sleep–wake disorder. It is fairly common in Alzheimer's sufferers. Their internal circadian clock has become completely disassociated from any semblance of a normal sleep–wake schedule. The best treatment is plenty of bright light exposure during the day along with structured activities. In some studies the addition of small doses of melatonin at night is reported to be helpful.

USE OF SEASONAL AFFECTIVE DISORDER (SAD) LAMP

Q. If someone wakes up every day at 11:00 a.m. and uses a SAD lamp for one hour, then goes to sleep at 3:00 a.m. in a room that is completely dark, will that person have the same health compared to if he would wake up at 5:00 a.m, use a SAD lamp for an hour, and go to sleep at 9:00 p.m.? So my question is . . . what, if anything, influences the body clock besides light and temperature of the body? Do the energy of the moon and sun and gravity affect the body, even if the room you sleep in is completely light-proof? Is sleep healthier at certain times, even if you sleep in a lightproof and soundproof room and use a SAD lamp immediately after you wake up?

A. What you are describing is someone with delayed sleep phase syndrome. As far as the health of the person who goes to bed at 3:00 a.m. and sleeps until 11:00 a.m., his or her health should be no different than the person with the more conventional sleep–wake cycle. The body clock is also affected by social and dietary influences such as the timing of meals. As for sunlight, if the room is dark and sunlight cannot strike the retina, there should be no influence.

JET LAG

Q. My wife and I are traveling to England this summer. We have had problems with jet lag before. How can we prevent this?

A. Since you are traveling east, you will be going to bed at a much earlier time than at home as far as your biological clock is concerned. It will take several days for your internal clock to adjust. I would advise that you progressively go to bed one hour earlier each day at home for three days, until you are going to bed three hours earlier. Expose yourself to bright sunlight upon awakening. This will help to reset your biological clock to an earlier sleep time at your destination.

SHIFT WORK DISORDER

Q. My fiancé has the WORST time sleeping of anyone I know. She works the night shift and lives with her mom. If her baby nephew comes over during the day and cries, she wakes up and can't sleep at all. She is constantly waking up covered in sweat even though she's not hot. Her dreams wake her up and she never feels like she is fully rested. She'll get off work super tired but cannot sleep for hours once she gets home. Melatonin hasn't helped. I feel so bad for her. Any advice would be appreciated.

A. Your fiancé has shift work disorder (SWD). Her bedroom needs to be very quiet. Consider white noise like a fan while sleeping or moving to a quieter bedroom. She should be wearing sunglasses, preferably blue blockers, on the drive home. No caffeine in the last three to four hours of her shift. On her days off, try to keep her sleep–wake schedule close to her days on. Finally, I am a bit bothered by the bad dreams and sweating. That could be a sign of sleep apnea. If she continues to have these problems, a consultation with a sleep specialist would be a good idea.

USE OF SLEEP AIDS

Q. I recently started a job working three night shifts in a row. Do you have any ideas as to when to sleep so that I can function like a normal person the rest of the week? Would it be safe to take a sleep aid when I know I have to work?

A. My first thought is, are you experiencing problems? Approximately 10% of shift workers have trouble as evidenced by an inability to stay awake at work or trouble falling asleep upon returning home. Add to that increased irritability and difficulty concentrating—then you have what we call SWD.

The key to dealing with this problem is exposing oneself to bright light during the first five to six hours of the night shift, and then scrupulously avoiding light on the way home. Dark glasses and a visor can be very useful. Melatonin taken upon arriving home may help one to sleep. The bedroom must be dark and family members need to keep the noise level down. A one- to two-hour nap in the evening before work is helpful. Most importantly, if this is a long-term job, you must try to adhere to the schedule as much as possible, even on your days off. If you follow these guidelines, you may be able to get your biological clock aligned with your new sleep–wake schedule.

LACK OF SLEEP CAUSING ILLNESS?

Q. My husband is always getting sick. He gets at least three colds a year and has had pneumonia twice in the last three years. His doctor can find no obvious cause. He sleeps no more than six hours a night and is a shift worker. Is it possible that his lack of sleep can be a cause of his frequent illnesses?

A. This is a great question. The answer is yes. Based on recent studies, we know that lack of sleep inhibits the production of antiviral antibodies. Even more impressive is that following vaccinations for viruses, such as hepatitis B or influenza, insufficient sleep leads to a weaker response to the vaccine. Finally, the incidence of infections in shift workers who have trouble sleeping is significantly higher than in the general population.

DIFFICULTY STAYING AWAKE ON THE JOB

Q. I have been moved to the night shift at my factory. It has been four months now and I am finding it very hard to stay awake on the job. I go to sleep as soon as I get home and sleep seven to eight hours. Despite that, I am having trouble staying awake. In this economy, I can't afford to lose my job. Would you have any ideas?

A. Yes, talk to your doctor about this. The FDA has approved the medications Provigil and Nuvigil for shift workers with your problem. I would consider this as an option until you either adapt to the night shift or you return to the day shift.

TROUBLE GETTING TO SLEEP AFTER SHIFT

Q. My employer has put me on the night shift. I'm having a difficult time getting to sleep in the morning. It can take me three or more hours to fall asleep, and then I have a really hard time getting through the night. Do you have any suggestions to help me?

A. You are experiencing what most shift workers go through initially. Your internal, what we call *circadian clock*, is out of phase with your new environment. There are things that you can do to hasten adaptation. First, wear dark glasses home in the morning. Exposure to sunlight will only make it more difficult to fall asleep. Second, try melatonin upon returning home and going to sleep. Melatonin will not only help you get to sleep but will speed up adaptation by your circadian clock. Last, try to stay close to your new sleep–wake schedule even on your days off.

MEDICATIONS TO STAY AWAKE

Q. I recently started working a night shift job. This is my first nighttime position and, after two months, I am still having trouble staying awake on the job. I cannot afford to lose this job. Friends tell me there are medications that might help. Is this true?

A. Yes, there are currently two medications approved by the FDA for shift workers. They are Provigil and Nuvigil. Both medications are wakefulness-promoting agents. However, other measures, such as a two-hour nap before the shift, judicious use of caffeine early in the shift, and exposure to bright light may help. Also, try to stay up later on your days off.

STAYING ALERT

Q. I was switched to the night shift at my factory. I am having a hard time staying alert while on the job. I started drinking coffee all night but then I can't stay asleep the following day when I need my sleep. Is there anything that can be done to help my situation?

A. Yes, what you are experiencing is a very common problem in people working the night shift. However, there are some potential solutions. First, try taking a one- or two-hour nap just before going to work. Second, it's okay to drink coffee, but limit it to no more than one cup at the beginning of the shift. In fact, this combined with a prework nap has been found to be more effective than either alone. Finally, if all else fails, speak to your doctor about the medications that have been approved by the FDA for excessive sleepiness and can help shift workers to stay alert and awake at work.

IMPACT OF AGE ON STAYING AWAKE

Q: I am 57 years old and for years I have worked as the night manager of a supermarket. I work four 10-hour shifts and then I am off for three days. For the last few years, I have had more trouble staying awake at work, as well as sleeping at home. Would you have any ideas?

A: As we age, our ability to do night shift work becomes increasingly more difficult. On average, after the age of 50, our circadian clock tends to shift to an earlier sleep time, making night shift work more difficult. I would recommend you wear dark glasses on your way home from work. Your bedroom should be dark. The use of blackout blinds is helpful. At work, try to be in a well-lit environment at least for the first half of your shift. A brief power nap (less than 45 minutes) one hour prior to work may help. In addition, a 30-minute nap at work might be beneficial. On your days off you should try to adhere to the same schedule as you have at work.

Self-Check: Self-Assessment for Night Owls and Morning Larks: Delayed Sleep-Phase Syndrome versus Advanced Sleep-Phase Disorder

The original questionnaire was first published in 1976 as the Horne–Ostberg test. The shortened version that follows reveals whether you function better toward the end of a day or at the beginning of one.

For each question, choose the one response that best describes you. When complete, add up the score for each response. The final score will give you some indication of whether you are more of a person of the morning or of the evening.

Breakfast: How is your appetite in the first half-hour after you wake up in the morning?

1 ____ Very poor

2 ____ Fairly good

3 ____ Fairly good

4 ____ Very good

How do you feel for the first half-hour after you wake up in the morning?

1 ____ Very tired

2 ____ Fairly tired

3 ____ Fairly refreshed

4 ____ Very refreshed

When you have no commitments the next day, at what time do you go to bed compared to your usual bedtime?

4 ____ Seldom or never later

3 ____ Less than one hour later

2 ____ One to two hours later

1 ____ More than two hours later

You are staring a new fitness regime. A friend suggests joining his fitness class between 7:00 a.m. and 8:00 a.m. How do you think you'd perform?

4 ____ Would be in good form

3 ____ Would be in reasonable form

2 ___ Would find it difficult

1 ___ Would find it very difficult

At what time in the evening do you feel tired and need sleep?

5 ___ 8:00 p.m. to 9:00 p.m.

4 ___ 9:00 p.m. to 10:15 p.m.

3 ___ 10:15 p.m. to 12:45 a.m.

2 ___ 12:45 a.m. to 2:00 a.m.

1 ___ 2:00 a.m. to 3:00 a.m.

If you went to bed at 11:00 p.m., how tired would you be?

0 ___ Not at all tired

2 ___ A little tired

3 ___ Fairly tired

5 ___ Very tired

One night you have to remain awake between 4:00 a.m. and 6:00 a.m. You have no commitments the next day. Which suits you best?

1 ___ Not to go to bed until 6:00 a.m.

2 ___ Nap before 4:00 a.m. and after 6:00 a.m.

3 ___ Sleep before 4:00 a.m. and nap after 6:00 a.m.

4 ___ Sleep before 4:00 a.m. and remain awake after 6:00 a.m.

At what time of day do you feel your best?

5 ___ 5:00 a.m. to 8:00 a.m.

4 ___ 8:00 a.m. to 10:00 a.m.

3 ___ 10:00 a.m. to 5:00 p.m.

2 ___ 5:00 p.m. to 10:00 p.m.

1 ___ 10:00 p.m. to 5:00 a.m.

Do you think of yourself as a morning or evening person?

6 ___ Morning type

4 ___ More morning type than evening type

2 ___ More evening type than morning type

0 ___ Evening type

Suppose that you can choose your own work hours, but you have to work five hours per day. When would you like to START your working day?

5 ___ 4:00 a.m. to 8:00 a.m.

4 ___ 8:00 a.m. to 9:00 a.m.

3 ___ 9:00 a.m. to 2:00 p.m.

2 ___ 2:00 p.m. to 5:00 p.m.

1 ___ 5:00 p.m. to 4:00 a.m.

SCORING

1. Add up the number of points that you scored for each answer.
2. The maximum number of points you have from this questionnaire is 46 and the minimum is 8.
3. The higher your score, you are more of a lark that functions better in the morning.
4. The lower your score, you are more of a night owl that functions better in the evening.
5. The majority of people come somewhere between these two extremes.

7

No Sleeping with Apnea

Laugh and the world laughs with you, snore and you sleep alone.

—ANTHONY BURGESS

While there are differing types of sleep disorders, only a few are part of the common vernacular. One of them is sleep apnea. You may associate it with snoring. Sleep apnea is a chronic sleep condition in which breathing repeatedly stops and starts. An apnea is a complete cessation of airflow, while a hypopnea is a reduction in airflow accompanied by either a drop in blood oxygen level or an arousal from sleep. There are two types of sleep apnea, which are different in their symptoms and require different treatments. The more common type is obstructive sleep apnea, and the less common is central sleep apnea.

Most bed partners might call the first symptom of apnea the loud snoring that keeps them awake. The silence of suspended breathing would be a more telling symptom of apnea. Not everyone who snores has sleep apnea, but those who do are at risk not only for diminished quality of life, but also for life-threatening conditions including stroke, heart attack, and diabetes.

Moreover, others' sleep apnea could be a threat to your own life if they are behind a wheel and have not adhered to treatments. The following stories are not rare. In fact, nearly every day you can read or see news about a car veering off the road, 18-wheelers sliding into cars, or school buses full of children swerving in traffic. The news always reports how many cars were damaged, how many homes were evacuated due to toxic spills, how many people died and were injured, but you rarely learn why the event happened. The following four incidents are not anomalies, but quite common:

- In 2008, Train 533 of the Canadian National/Illinois Central Railway was heading south around dawn and the engineer failed to see or stop at the glowing red stop light. The conductor also failed to see the flashing red light and did not warn the engineer that he had passed it. Meantime, train 243 was clipping along northbound on the same track. Both locomotives with loaded box-cars snaking behind them smashed head-on into each other. The National Transportation Safety Board (NTSB) reported, ". . . probable cause . . . was the train 533 crew members' fatigue . . . primarily due to the engineer's untreated and the conductor's insufficiently treated obstructive sleep apneas."
- In 2008, in Hawaii, island-hopping passengers of Flight 1002 left Honolulu airport on time and expected to land at Hilo within the hour. Instead, the plane flew over the island, over the next two islands, and headed toward the watery horizon. Only one pilot was diagnosed with sleep apnea, yet both fell asleep. "Both pilots unintentionally

fell asleep during cruise flight. The Safety Board received information after the accident that one of the pilots was diagnosed with obstructive sleep apnea, which, without medical treatment, is associated with reduced sleep."

- In 2008, a refrigerated Volvo semitrailer headed east on I-44 at 69 miles per hour with the cruise control on. The truck driver failed to slow down or brake and collided full force with a long line of cars that were slowing or stopped. The NTSB summarized the cause as, "driver's fatigue, caused by the combined effects of acute sleep loss, circadian disruption associated with his shift work schedule, and mild sleep apnea, which resulted in the driver's failure to react to slowing and stopped traffic ahead by applying the brakes or performing any evasive maneuver to avoid colliding with the traffic queue."
- In 2011, the NTSB attributed a collision between two BNSF Railway freight trains in Red Oak, Iowa, to the "failure of the crew of the striking train to comply with the signal indication requiring them to operate in accordance with restricted speed requirements and stop short of the standing train because they had fallen asleep due to fatigue resulting from their irregular work schedules and their medical conditions."

Sleep apnea is a serious problem. Current estimates show that 18 million Americans have sleep apnea. This number has doubled since the early 1990s and survey results attribute the increase to the rising incidence of obesity in the United States. Sadly, 80% of these people are undiagnosed and untreated.

It is important to diagnose and treat this disorder. The health risks of untreated sleep apnea are substantial. A recent study showed that if untreated, people with severe sleep apnea were 25% more likely to die over a 10-year period than those who did not have the disease.

However, this sleep disorder is treatable, with good results. It's been reported that treating sleep apnea resulted in a 52% drop in motor vehicle accidents, a 49% decrease in heart attacks, and a 31% decrease in stroke in those with moderate to severe disease over a 10-year period. How I wish the train engineer and conductor, the pilots, and the truck driver had received treatment!

Obstructive Sleep Apnea (OSA)

Obstructive Sleep Apnea is a common disorder affecting at least 2% to 4% of the adult population. The closing or obstruction of the airway is the defining trait of OSA. Most people experience pauses in breathing while they sleep. For people with sleep apnea, these pauses occur more often, and sometimes as often as once or twice each minute. Other symptoms of apnea include the telltale snoring, shallow breathing, as well as a choking or snorting sound whenever the person awakens (because they are not breathing!) The symptoms and subsequent consequences of OSA are the result of the repetitive collapse of the upper airway that obstructs breathing.

The upper airway is not a rigid structure. Its ability to stay open depends upon a balance of forces. Normal muscle activity that contributes to keeping the airway open relaxes when we go to sleep. If the airway is smaller to begin with because of fat deposits, anatomy, or more frequently in the case of children, enlarged tonsils and adenoids, the airway is more likely to collapse while you sleep.

The other contributing factor is the force exerted to inhale at night. The more forceful the effort, the more negative the pressure in the upper airway. This contributes to collapse, especially during sleep when the opposing dilator muscles are not at full strength. That is why sleep apnea may worsen with nasal congestion and is more likely in mouth breathers.

Finally, alcohol and many of the commonly prescribed sleep aids can weaken the upper airway muscles during sleep. This further promotes the collapse and sleep apnea.

HOW THE BODY WORKS ON OSA

- When you fall asleep, the upper airway muscles relax. You lose the ability to control their strength.
- If you have an airway with a smaller diameter, then you are more likely to experience collapse and obstructed breathing when you fall asleep.
- Factors such as obesity, large tonsils, or a backward positioned jaw can result in a smaller airway.
- In addition, alcohol and certain medications can further weaken the muscles when you are asleep.

SLEEP APNEA, HYPERTENSION, AND STROKE

Phil's cardiologist sent him to me. Phil had an irregular heartbeat, called atrial fibrillation, that he most frequently noticed upon waking in the morning. Phil is 59 years old, relatively healthy with no underlying medical problems, but he keeps going into atrial fibrillation. He had already been to the emergency room and admitted on two occasions. The attending physician used cardioversion to reset his heart rhythm electrically, back to its regular pattern.

For some reason, Phil kept going back into atrial fib. Finally, his cardiologist asked him, "Well, do you snore?"

"My wife says my snoring is not loud, so it isn't a big deal."

"Phil, it could be a big deal because we now know that a very common cause of atrial fibrillation is sleep apnea. On top of that, we also know that after cardioversion, if we don't treat the sleep apnea, up to 50% of patients will go back into the atrial fibrillation."

When Phil arrived in my office, I observed a beefy, overweight, middle-aged man. He was a little skeptical, asking, "Well, how come I'm not sleepy? How come I don't feel tired?"

"You know, Phil, we don't know yet that you have sleep apnea, but I certainly suspect it, based upon your history of morning awakenings with atrial fib and your snoring. What you might find interesting is that several studies show that cardiac patients with sleep apnea tend not to present with sleepiness. That means that the sympathetic nervous system is on overdrive, which may be part of the problems with cardiac patients to begin with. Therefore, your alerting system is in overdrive all day long, so you tend not to get sleepy. Frequently, the first inkling we have of sleep apnea is when you go into atrial fibrillation or you have your first heart attack."

Phil listened, nodded, and was willing to seriously consider the recommendation put to him by his cardiologist and me. He went to the sleep study, and found he had sleep apnea. Actually he has a significant sleep apnea, which means he stops breathing 30 to 40 times an hour.

Believe it or not, during one of those episodes, he had a short run of atrial fibrillation, which went away. I've seen that happen before. When Phil returned to see me, I was able to show him on the computer, "Here you are. You stopped breathing. We even have you going into a short burst of atrial fibrillation at the end of one of your apneas."

He stared and shook his head, not in denial, but more like, wow!

"Phil, I said, "you are lucky your cardiologist referred you to me. Most cardiac patients don't seek out any help because they're not sleepy. Unfortunately, the first time I see them is when they have an event."

"I am lucky, Doc. I appreciate knowing. Now I can get some help."

The autonomic nervous system consists of the "fight or flight" sympathetic nervous system and the parasympathetic nervous system. Normally, when we go to sleep, the calming parasympathetic nervous system predominates and our blood pressure drops an average of 10 points. However, in people with sleep apnea, there is a stimulation of the sympathetic nervous system during sleep. This is in response to the low oxygen levels that accompany the respiratory events in conjunction with the stress response brought on by the effort to breathe against a closed airway. This results in surges of blood pressure as high as 240 mmHg at the termination of each of these events. Therefore, people with sleep apnea lose the normal drop in blood pressure with sleep. In fact, their blood pressure may skyrocket. Eventually, this nocturnal elevation spills over into the daytime and results in persistent hypertension. This, as well as other factors we will go into in the following questions and answers, results in end organ damage to the heart and brain. In part, because of this, recent studies have shown the incidence of sleep apnea in heart attack and stroke victims to be over 50%.

THIS IS YOUR BRAIN ON SLEEP APNEA

In addition to the other health risks, sleep apnea can also wreak havoc with your brain. Using a combination magnetic resonance imaging (MRI) and voxel-based morphometry (VBM), researchers have determined that patients with untreated sleep apnea have decreased gray matter over several regions of the brain. These areas, including the hippocampus and frontal lobes, control several executive functions, including skills in planning, working memory, attention span, problem solving, verbal reasoning, and multitasking. Perhaps this is why people with sleep apnea are sometimes misdiagnosed with early onset Alzheimer's.

Sleep apnea has also been associated with emotional disorders, including anxiety, PTSD, obsessive-compulsive disorder, and panic disorders. The research in this area began when physicians began noticing a high rate of coexistence between these disorders and sleep apnea. Given the statistics, they knew it had to be more than a coincidence; however, it was years before they could figure out the connection.

Recent studies indicate that sleep apnea is the cause of these disorders, not the other way around. In addition to gray matter, apnea also affects the brain's limbic system. One of the functions of the limbic system is to regulate the endocrine system, including stress hormones. An increase of these hormones can trigger the sympathetic nervous system, higher levels of anxiety, and even the "fight or flight" response to external stimuli. In addition, sleep apnea also interrupts the stages of sleep, particularly REM (rapid eye movement). The REM stage is the time when one processes the stressful events they experienced during the day; therefore, when REM is continually interrupted, the patient misses out on the opportunity to purge him- or herself of trauma. This also increases stress hormones, and after an extended period, creates the secondary emotional disorder.

SLEEP APNEA AND DIABETES

A study presented at the 2013 American Thoracic Society International Conference demonstrated that in people with prediabetes, treatment of associated sleep apnea improved blood sugar control. Two weeks of treatment with continuous positive airway pressure (CPAP) resulted in a significant lowering of blood sugar.

We have known for several years that there is a link between diabetes and sleep apnea. Sleep apnea is a stress-producing condition occurring while a person is asleep. It results in high levels of cortisol and activation of the sympathetic nervous system. This can result in significant elevations in blood sugar. At the same time, it is also ruining your oxygen levels. This causes the release of substances called inflammatory mediators, which inhibit the ability of insulin to get into the cells. This is referred to as insulin resistance. In response, the pancreas, where insulin is produced, attempts to put out more and more insulin. However, there comes a time when it can no longer do this, and that is when prediabetes becomes diabetes.

We know that the incidence of sleep apnea in diabetics is high. Previously it was felt that obesity, which is common to both conditions, was the link. However, now it is becoming increasingly clear that sleep apnea may be the cause of diabetes in those who suffer from this breathing disorder.

So what are the implications? First, weight loss is extremely important and can improve both diabetes and sleep apnea. However, if you have been diagnosed with early diabetes and snore loudly or are constantly sleepy or fatigued, you may have sleep apnea. In this case, bringing it to the attention of your health care provider could result not only in an improvement in how you feel but also in your blood sugar control.

CHILDREN AND SLEEP APNEA

We often think of OSA as an ailment of the middle-aged and elderly. Yet it can affect anyone, even children. The causes of OSA are different for kids, as compared to adults, such as enlarged tonsils or adenoids. The symptoms, however, are often the same in children and adults: snoring, sleepiness during the day, trouble paying attention, and even behavioral issues. However, unlike adults, many children exhibit hyperactivity. In fact, many children with OSA are mistakenly diagnosed with attention deficit hyperactivity disorder (ADHD).

The most common treatment is surgery—either a tonsillectomy or adenoidectomy. Some children are prescribed a CPAP machine, or in the case of childhood obesity, placed on a weight loss regimen.

SYMPTOMS

Do you experience these symptoms during the day?

1. Sleepy
2. Foggy
3. Forgetful
4. Depressed
5. Anxious
6. Mood disorder

During the day, those with sleep apnea may feel sleepy, foggy, or forgetful. They may also experience depression and anxiety that rise to the level of a mood disorder. Women with OSA typically have more daytime sleepiness, anxiety, depression, and reduced quality of sleep. Researchers attribute this to structural changes in the brain, specifically the white matter, caused by sleep apnea.

Do you experience any of the following at night?

1. You experience a higher than normal incidence of pauses in breathing while you sleep, whether four or five times an hour or as frequently as once or twice a minute.
2. When you start breathing again, it's with a loud snort or choking sound.
3. You urinate several times during the night.
4. You experience sexual difficulties.

You would recognize these symptoms if you suspect that you or another has OSA:

Frequent Nighttime Urination

Sleep apnea is commonly associated with frequent nighttime urination. How this happens has only recently been understood. When someone has an episode of apnea, an effort to breathe against a closed airway occurs. This results in the development of profound negative pressure in the chest cavity. Consequently, the heart, especially the small chambers called atria that sit atop the muscular chambers called ventricles, are stretched. When these chambers are stretched, they respond by putting out a hormone called atrial natriuretic peptide. This hormone is a diuretic. That means it induces an increase of urine. You see, the heart is not that smart. When stretched, it interprets the stretching as too much fluid in the body. This is an appropriate response when dealing with heart failure, but is a nuisance when the cause is OSA. The good news is that when the obstruction to breathing is reversed, the nighttime urination comes to an abrupt end.

Sexual Dysfunction

The connection between sleep apnea and sexual dysfunction is well–documented, and all the studies have historically focused on men. Definitely, sleep apnea relates to erectile dysfunction (ED) and also to sexual dysfunction. The prevalence of men with sleep apnea who also have ED is as high as 40%. The reasons for this problem appear to be twofold. In some men, sleep apnea can cause low testosterone levels. In others, repetitive drops in oxygen cause a problem with the ability of small blood vessels to supply adequate blood flow to the penis. This is called endothelial dysfunction and is very common in sleep apnea. The good news is that the majority of men afflicted with sleep apnea will show significant improvement in sexual function when their sleep apnea is treated.

More recently, however, doctors have found that women suffering from OSA also experience sexual difficulties, including problems involving desire, arousal, orgasm, pain, vaginal lubrication, and sexual satisfaction. In fact, studies have shown that between 34% and 54% of women with sleep apnea also experience female sexual dysfunction (FSD). Like men, the severity of the sexual symptoms are in direct correlation with the apnea itself, specifically, the drops in oxygen that occur during the "pauses" in breathing. When the oxygen gets low enough, the person takes a breath, thus bringing up the oxygen level again. This yo-yoing cause is known as oxidative stress; it introduces free oxygen radicals, which can damage nerve tissues, as well as the lining of our blood vessels. That puts women with sleep apnea at a much higher risk of stroke and heart attack. For women, the destruction of these nerve endings also affects sexuality, hence the FSD.

Men with OSA often have low testosterone. This does not seem to factor into sexual dysfunction in women. Studies show that levels of estrogen, progesterone, and testosterone are the same in women with sleep apnea, whether they have FSD or not.

Women experiencing sexual dysfunction should definitely tell their health care providers that they would like to be tested for sleep apnea. The good news is that once the sleep apnea is treated, the FSD usually disappears.

TREATMENT OPTIONS

The best way to diagnose sleep apnea is by visiting a special sleep clinic. The patient spends the night at the clinic, while trained sleep specialists monitor his or her breathing, heart rate and other vitals. (There are home monitors that gauge these things, but they are not as effective.)

Once it is determined that you do have sleep apnea, your doctor will characterize its severity based on several factors, including how often these breathing pauses occur, how low your oxygen drops during these pauses, and how sleepy you feel during waking hours.

Continuous Positive Airway Pressure (CPAP)

The most commonly prescribed, and most thoroughly researched treatment for OSA is a CPAP machine. The machine pushes a constant stream of air through a mask that keeps the throat and airway open. There are different kinds of masks; some fit over the nose, while others fit over both the nose and mouth. For effective treatment, the patient must use the machine every night, and most likely for the rest of his or her life. A patient can choose to cure their sleep apnea through some other means (surgery or weight loss). However, researchers noticed marked improvement after three months of using CPAP, with restoration of gray matter lost as a result of the sleep apnea.

CPAP treatment can also help with OSA's assault on the limbic system; however, it may take some time, especially if the coexisting disorder has taken on a life of its own. This often leads to a vicious cycle. After beginning treatment, patients may still experience light sleeping, claustrophobia, and shortness of breath, which only makes the CPAP machine—with its mask that covers the nose and/or mouth—even less appealing. This is especially true for returning veterans with PTSD, who are statistically the less likely to adhere to treatment. Still, I have found that with continued treatment, patients will experience a very noticeable improvement over time. Often a willingness on the part of the physician to explain both the long-term benefits and the expected initial problems is extremely helpful in getting the patient to comply.

Mandibular Advancement Device (MAD)

This is a mouthpiece—usually made of hard plastic—that covers the upper and lower teeth. Like the CPAP, there are several different kinds of MADs. Some hold the tongue in place, keep the jaw forward, and the airway open.

Positive Airway Pressure Nap (PAP-NAP)

Dr. Barry Krakow of New Mexico pioneered PAP-NAP, a daytime approach to help patients who are anxious or claustrophobic or have difficulty using the CPAP approach. The patient works personally with a sleep technologist through coaching, relaxation, use of imagery, desensitization, and deeper breathing while being exposed to various masks and forms of pressure delivery for achieving CPAP compliance. Patients can nap during therapy. This is a novel approach to acclimating people to the usage of positive airway devices for sleep apnea. In my sleep centers we have found it to be an invaluable tool in achieving compliance.

Hypoglossal Nerve Stimulator

A hypoglossal nerve stimulator (HGNS) is an implantable electronic device that acts like a pacemaker. It stimulates the hypoglossal nerve during inhalation. This in turn stimulates the muscles of the tongue resulting in protrusion and opening of the airway during sleep. It is very close to being released as a treatment for OSA.

Weight Loss

Since obesity is often a factor in OSA, it stands to reason that with substantial weight loss, one can often lessen the severity of the OSA or, in some cases, cure it altogether. The measures one takes to lose the excess weight depends on several factors, including lifestyle and how much weight they need to lose. Some combine diet and exercise, while others undergo bariatric surgery.

Uvulopalatopharyngoplasty

Uvulopalatopharyngoplasty (UPPP or UP3) is a surgical procedure to make the airway wider. The doctor removes excess tissue, whether it is the uvula (the soft tissue that hangs down from the back of the throat), part of the soft palate (at the roof of the mouth), or the tonsils and/or adenoids; the doctor may even remove part of the tongue if he/she determines it is contributing to the apnea. This surgery has received mixed reactions from the medical community. In addition to the usual risks that accompany surgery, UPPP does not always work. Worse yet, it sometimes appears to have been successful when in fact it wasn't. In other words, the patient may stop snoring, but is still experiencing those dangerous pauses in breathing. This means he or she still has sleep apnea that requires treatment. In fact, many patients still need to use CPAP after undergoing UPPP.

Central Sleep Apnea (CSA)

Central Sleep Apnea occurs when your breathing repeatedly stops for 10 seconds or longer because the brain's respiratory control center fails to send a signal to the respiratory system to breathe.

Why does this happen? Think in terms of what would cause a break in communication between the brain stem and the body. Possibilities include tumors, strokes, opioid medications, or influences such as neurological disorders.

Breathing stops numerous times throughout the night with no visible effort to breathe followed by:

1. A drop in oxygen
2. A rise in carbon dioxide
3. A brief arousal from sleep in order to take a breath

Normally, when you go to sleep, carbon dioxide levels increase because your breathing is shallow and your respiratory rate drops. While asleep, the respiratory center shuts down if carbon dioxide levels drop to slightly lower than normal wakefulness levels. This level, called the apneic threshold, lasts until the carbon dioxide amount rises to normal sleep levels. People with CSA tend to have an unstable respiratory center that responds excessively to the return of elevated carbon dioxide. They then hyperventilate and again drop carbon dioxide levels below the apneic threshold, resulting in another central apnea.

There are two major forms of CSA:

● **Primary CSA** is a form of sleep apnea that has no underlying medical condition or medication causing it. It is rare, occurring in about 5% of all cases of sleep apnea.

● **Secondary CSA** is more common with several types.

   ▪ **Cheyne-Stokes breathing** refers to a cyclic pattern of breathing and is most common in people who have experienced a stroke or have weak hearts. As an observer, you would see a person demonstrate periods of increasingly deeper breathing that would reach a peak in 30 to 60 seconds, followed by a decline in the depth of respirations. After 30 to 60 seconds of this decline comes a complete absence of breathing for at least 10 seconds. This is the apnea, after which the whole pattern tends to occur repeatedly during the night.

   ▪ **CSA caused by the use of pain medications of the opioid family** like morphine, methadone, oxycodone, and hydrocodone. In some studies, as much as 40% of the patients on methadone programs to stay off heroin, are experiencing this type of CSA. The accompanying sedatives and sleeping pills frequently given to these patients can exacerbate it.

- **Complex sleep apnea** is a form of sleep apnea in which central apneas persist or emerge during attempts to treat OSA with a CPAP or bi-level BiPAP device. I is more common at higher altitudes of mountainous regions.

The good news for persons diagnosed with CSA is that once diagnosed, all of these forms of CSA can be treated. In some patients, it may be as simple as supplemental oxygen at night. In other patients, improving cardiac function or getting off opioids when possible may eliminate the problem.

However, in cases where this is not possible, sleep medicine has some sophisticated machines to deal with the problem. Recently, an adaptive servo ventilation device was approved by most insurers and Medicare for this condition. The unit is not much larger than a CPAP machine and takes care of both the OSA and central apneas. Unlike CPAP machines, if it senses an absence of an effort to breathe (a central apnea), it can generate timed back-up breaths until the person begins to initiate a breath on his or her own.

Answers to Your Questions

DIFFERENCE BETWEEN CSA AND OSA

Q. For several years I have been having trouble staying awake. My doctor sent me for a sleep study and told me I had CSA. How is that different from the more common OSA?

A. In CSA, the person makes no effort to breathe during the event. The brain's respiratory center does not send any signals to the respiratory system to breathe. This results in arousals from sleep and poor sleep due to low oxygen levels. There are many causes for CSA. Sleep experts see it in patients on large doses of narcotics, in patients with weak hearts, and in those who have suffered from strokes in the past. In addition, a significant number of people have no underlying cause whatsoever.

TEEN'S BREATHING PATTERN IS APNEA?

Q. My 17-year-old son appears to sleep soundly. However, I have noticed that he usually takes three deep breaths at a fast rate, followed by no breathing for 7 to 10 seconds. Then the pattern repeats. He does not snore or gasp for air. He is overweight and I worry that he has sleep apnea.

A. From what you are describing, this could be a form of sleep apnea called CSA, which is caused by an intermittent failure of the ventilatory control center in the brain to signal the respiratory system to breathe. There are two important issues about your son. Does he have any symptoms during the day such as sleepiness, irritability, or trouble concentrating? In addition, does this go on throughout the night or just as he is falling asleep? If the latter, it may be normal, as central apneas are normal during our transition from wake to sleep.

SLEEP APNEA AND CHILDREN

Q. Is it true that if untreated in children, sleep apnea can lead to problems? My grandson is nine years old and when he sleeps over he snores like a freight train and I think he stops breathing. My daughter thinks I'm being an alarmist and there is no need to be concerned. What do you think?

A. I cannot tell you if your grandson has sleep apnea, but I can tell you that the American Academy of Pediatrics recommends a thorough evaluation for sleep apnea in children who snore chronically. I can also tell you that a recent study published in the journal *Sleep*, showed that children with moderate sleep apnea had significant elevations of blood pressure during apneic events while sleeping. This was especially noted during REM (dream) sleep. The authors feel that since elevated blood pressure in childhood predicts adult hypertension, this should be addressed as early as possible. Another recent study showed a high incidence of depression in children with OSA.

Q. My eight-year-old daughter snores loudly. I took her to see an ENT (ear, nose, and throat) specialist who advised we have her tonsils and adenoids removed. My pediatrician said we should first get a sleep study performed. What do you think?

A. I agree with your pediatrician for several reasons. First, before performing any surgery, you want to know if it is necessary. In the absence of sleep apnea, it might not be indicated. Second, if your child has severe sleep apnea, postoperative respiratory complications are more common, and precautions such as overnight monitoring after the surgery are indicated. Finally, if the sleep apnea is severe, a repeat test after surgery is necessary in most cases to confirm it has been cured.

SLEEP APNEA AND DEMENTIA

Q. My 74-year-old mom was diagnosed with early dementia. She has been having problems with her memory and can never remember where she puts things. She snores and her new neurologist wants to do a sleep study on her.

He says that sleep apnea can be the cause of some of her issues. Is this true?

A. Yes it is. It is not uncommon for sleep apnea, especially in the elderly, to present with problems using memory and focusing. In fact, a particular area of the brain involved in memory called the hippocampus is very likely to be damaged by low oxygen levels associated with sleep apnea. I would advise you to urge your mom to be tested. If positive, there could be a significant improvement in her mental status.

APNEA AND BLOOD SUGAR

Q. My doctor recently ran some blood tests on me and found that I am prediabetes. I snore loudly and she told me that if I have sleep apnea, treating it might improve my blood sugar. Is this true?

A. Yes, several studies have shown that treatment of sleep apnea improves blood sugar control in diabetes and prediabetes. Sleep apnea causes insulin resistance and in most studies insulin resistance improved within two weeks of treatment.

CPAP

Q. I have severe sleep apnea and have been on CPAP for three months. I don't feel any better now than I did before. What do you think?

A. First, you need to be sure that your machine is working effectively. Most machines come with a downloadable smart card. Your physician should be able to review it and tell if your sleep apnea is being successfully treated. Second, not all people placed on CPAP will "feel better." Up to 10% of those treated may continue to feel sleepy and fatigued. However, they are still getting the same benefit in terms of stroke and heart attack reduction that the other 90% get. So make sure it is working effectively and stick with it.

Q. I was recently diagnosed with sleep apnea and I use a CPAP machine every night. I am very obese and have read that if I lose a lot of weight I will no longer need to use the CPAP. Is that true?

A. It is possible that you will not need the CPAP. It depends on how severe, how many times you stop breathing per hour, and how much weight you lose. I can tell you that after bariatric surgery, approximately 60% of patients with sleep apnea no longer require CPAP. The good news is that weight loss is much easier after the treatment of sleep apnea. If you do lose a lot of weight you probably should be retested to see if you still have the sleep disorder. Don't make the mistake of just stopping treatment because you think it is no longer necessary. Unfortunately, I am frequently referred patients who mistakenly made this assumption.

APNEA AND EPILEPSY

Q. My 52-year-old brother has epilepsy. He is on three medications but still has frequent seizures. According to his wife he was diagnosed with sleep apnea but rarely wears his CPAP mask. Could the sleep apnea have anything to do with his seizures?

A. Yes, the incidence of sleep apnea in refractory epilepsy is 30% to 40%, shown in several studies. Treating the sleep apnea results in a 50% decrease in seizures in most and a reduction in the number of anti-epileptic drugs required.

THE DIFFERENCE BETWEEN CPAP AND ADAPTO SERVO VENTILATION (ASV)

Q. I had a sleep study done last month, and I have a form of sleep apnea referred to as CSA. The report that my doctor received said that I should return to the lab for treatment of this condition. They recommended a machine called an ASV. My doctor explained the difference between a CPAP and an ASV, but I didn't understand. Could you please explain?

A. In CSA, you periodically make no attempt to breathe during the night. CPAP machines are designed to work on the obstructive form of the disease. They splint the airway open with pressure to prevent it from collapsing. However, the CPAP machine cannot respond to a failure to make any effort to breathe. The ASV machines will sense this absence of effort and cycle in and breathe for you when this happens. They are specifically designed for CSA.

WHAT IS COMPLEX SLEEP APNEA?

Q. I had a sleep study performed and was diagnosed with sleep apnea. I was then asked to return to the sleep lab for a second study to determine the level of CPAP required in order to treat this condition. I was surprised when a third study was requested. Apparently, I have what they call complex sleep apnea, which requires a different type of machine other than a CPAP. What is this condition and why couldn't they get it right in the first place?

A. Complex sleep apnea is a newly described form of sleep apnea. About 10% to 15% of patients, when placed on CPAP, have episodes in which they stop breathing and make no effort to breathe for 10 seconds or more. It is as if they forget to take a breath. These events are called CSAs, as opposed to the more common OSAs. Central apneas turn out to be just as disruptive to sleep as obstructive apneas and cannot be treated with CPAP alone.

There is a new form of treatment for complex sleep apnea called adaptive servo ventilation. Returning to the sleep lab is normal for a third study with this new device, which is a small unit that delivers pressure just as CPAP does. However, it eliminates both types of breathing-related sleep abnormalities—central and obstructive apneas. Most of the research on this new machine is from the Mayo Clinic. This is probably what you will be treated with when you return for your third study.

CSA AND METHADONE

Q. I have been on methadone for pain for several years. Recently I underwent a sleep study and was told I have CSA, probably due to the methadone. I don't understand why it has no effect on my breathing during the day. Can you explain?

A. Most patients' respiratory systems adapt to narcotics within four weeks. However, that is not the case concerning their breathing while asleep. Unfortunately, up to 40% of patients on methadone develop CSA. This may also be an undetected cause of persistent fatigue in these folks.

CPAP CAUSED CSA?

Q. I was recently diagnosed and treated for obstructive sleep apnea. They put me on a CPAP machine. However, I then developed central apnea. I was told that a failure to make any effort to breathe characterizes central apnea and that the treatment with CPAP caused this. I changed to a machine that can treat my central apneas as well. Why would a CPAP machine cause this to happen?"

A. This is a great question. What you are referring to is called complex sleep apnea. We believe there may be two mechanisms that cause this in some patients. One is a stretching of the lung by the positive pressure. This can elicit a reflex that depresses respiration. The other is a drop in carbon dioxide brought about by the CPAP machine. The brain does not like low carbon dioxide levels and will stop sending signals to the lungs to breathe until the carbon dioxide builds up again.

Self-Check: What Is Your Risk of OSA?: Stop Bang Questionnaire

Answer each question YES or NO

Snoring	**Do you snore loudly?** (Louder than talking or loud enough to be heard through closed doors.)	YES	NO
Tired	Do you often **feel tired, fatigued, or sleepy** during the daytime?	YES	NO
Observed	Has anyone observed you **stop breathing** during your sleep?	YES	NO
Pressure	Do you have or are you being treated for **high blood pressure?**	YES	NO
Body mass	Is your **body mass index** more than 35?*	YES	NO
Age	Are you older than **50 years**?	YES	NO
Neck size	Does your **neck measure** more than 16 inches/40 cm around? (Measure at Adam's apple.)	YES	NO
Gender	Is your **gender male?**	YES	NO

*To calculate your BMI visit www.bmi-calculator.net
Reprinted with permission from the American Society of Anesthesiologists.

Count the items you marked as YES and enter here _____

OSA—High Risk—Score is 5 to 8
OSA—Intermediate Risk—Score is 3 or 4
OSA—Low Risk—Score is 0 to 2

PART THREE

Parasomnias

Para, of Greek origin, refers to something amiss or irregular; *somia* refers to conditions of sleep. Parasomnias are sleep disorders that are intrusive to sleep and involve abnormal movements, behaviors, emotions, perceptions, or dreams. Parasomnias may occur during each sleep stage:

1. Non-rapid eye movement (non-REM) parasomnias tend to develop during the first half of the night. They are frequently associated with slow-wave sleep and are referred to as arousal parasomnias. These include confusional arousals, night terrors, and sleepwalking. The individual frequently shows an abrupt arousal from deep sleep when they occur, but the waking is not complete. The higher brain centers, such as the frontal lobes and prefrontal cortex, remain in a sleep state. The result is an absence of higher brain functions that control impulsivity, reasoning, judgment, and memory for past actions.
2. Rapid eye movement (REM) parasomnias, such as REM sleep behavior disorder, occur during REM sleep. REM sleep makes up about 20% of our sleep and tends to

increase during the second half of the night. People with REM parasomnias may have dreams of a violent nature and may punch, kick, tackle, or dive out of bed, causing injury to themselves or to a bed partner. Most of the time—but not always—the person can recall a dream if awakened.

8

Sleepwalking and Night Terrors

Sleep isn't a break from our lives. It's the missing third of the puzzle of what it means to be living.

—DAVID K. RANDALL

Sleepwalking, also known as somnambulism, is common in children. However, sleepwalking may persist into or begin in adulthood. Sleepwalkers arise from slow wave sleep (non-REM) and walk, sit up in bed, or do other activities that are usually performed during a state of full consciousness. Sleepwalking usually happens during the first third of the night when most slow wave sleep occurs.

Night terrors, a state of intense fear with a piercing scream or cry, sweating, and agitation, also typically occur in the early stages of sleep and may coexist with sleepwalking.

Sleepwalking

A sleepwalker may sit up or bolt from bed. He or she is unresponsive to conversation or commands, and may be quiet or agitated. The sleepwalker's eyes can be open, but glazed over and not seeing as an awake person. Though appearing to be awake, the sleepwalker remains asleep. In rare instances, a sleepwalker may be violent if startled awake. Episodes of sleepwalking can last from 10 to 30 minutes. Some patients can retain images after waking, but most have total amnesia of the event.

The sleepwalker's behavior can be benign like a young child wandering through the house and going back to bed, or involve more complex behaviors. One sleepwalking 11-year-old always went to the back door and tried to go outside. One night, he was successful in unlocking the door and walked into the yard. His mother wondered how he'd managed to unlock the door.

SLEEPWALKING IN CHILDREN

Sleepwalking is more prevalent in children, especially in preschoolers and children between the ages of 3 and 12. Most kids who sleepwalk occasionally do not have an underlying sleep disorder. Children simply have more slow-wave sleep. In other words, a six-year-old might have 40% slow-wave sleep, and a young adult might have 15% to 20%. The more slow-wave sleep, the more likely a child is to sleepwalk. In these cases, children usually have spontaneous resolution after puberty because slow-wave sleep decreases.

An effective treatment to curb sleepwalking is scheduled awakenings. First, the parent should observe approximately what time the sleepwalking usually occurs. Then, they are instructed to gently and briefly awaken the child 30 minutes earlier than when they sleepwalk. This interrupts their sleep in a loving way. Doing this for 25 to 30 days can eliminate sleepwalking for up to six months. I don't use medications with kids unless the sleepwalking is very frequent because the scheduled awakenings tend to work with persistent parents.

If the sleepwalking is frequent and doesn't resolve after scheduled awakenings, we would consider a sleep study to rule out sleep apnea, periodic limb movement, or even nocturnal seizures, which can be misinterpreted as sleepwalking. Insufficient sleep may also be a possibility. Children have more deep, slow-wave sleep when they are sleep-deprived and thus there is more potential for sleep-walking. This was the case with a recent patient. Carmelita, seven years old and thin, came to the sleep clinic because she was a sleepwalker. Her parents reported that she watched television until eleven o'clock at night and then got up for school at six o'clock in the morning. This seven-year-old should be getting at least eleven hours of sleep, not seven hours. She was sleep-deprived, which was causing her sleep-walking. Once Carmelita started going to bed by 8:00 p.m., her frequent sleepwalking ended.

If another disorder is the cause, such as sleep apnea, treatment for these disorders is generally effective at elimi-nating the sleepwalking. In one study of prepubescent chil-dren with repetitive sleepwalking and night terrors, the parasomnias disappeared after the children were treated for sleep breathing disorders (SBD), restless legs syndrome (RLS), and periodic leg movements. Treatment effects were maintained at three months and at six months.

SLEEPWALKING IN ADULTS

Adults who sleepwalk most often exhibited it as children. The persistence or onset of sleepwalking in adulthood is less com-mon than in children but it is more common than previously thought. According to a 2012 study conducted by the Stanford University School of Medicine, about 3.6% of U.S. adults— or upward of 8.4 million—are prone to sleepwalking. Adult sleepwalkers are more likely than children to turn violent. One cohort research project (2007–2011) involved 140 adult sleepwalkers who were evaluated and followed over time at the Sleep Disorders Clinic in Montpellier, France. Violent behavior in sleep was investigated in 95 of those adults. Psychological stress, strong positive emotions, and sleep deprivation triggered the onset and frequency of violence in almost 60% of the participants. Among the adults whose pattern continued from childhood, 58% experienced violent sleepwalking episodes.

Genetics may play a role. Thirty-eight percent of sleepwalkers have a first-generation relative who is also a sleepwalker. The pattern of inheritance was the least understood aspect until recently. Researchers assessed sleepwalking in four generations of one family. Thirteen members were not affected and nine were sleepwalkers. They determined that sleepwalking passes through generations via one chromosome. You can inherit it from only one parent but not every person who carries that chromosome will pass it forward. More research needs to be done in order to determine who is most at risk for experiencing sleepwalking.

Possible triggers include:

● Lack of sleep, sleep-deprivation
● Sleep apnea
● Restless legs syndrome
● Stress or anxiety
● Traumatic events or post-traumatic stress disorder
● Lithium
● Ambien
● Benzodiazepine sleeping pills such as Halcion, diazepam, and somewhat with Lunesta.
● Atypical antipsychotics such as olanzapine (Zyprexa), quetiapine (Seroquel), and Risperdal.

As with children, sleep apnea, RLS, or periodic limb movements are causes in adults. By successfully treating these issues, the sleepwalking will diminish and disappear. My patient Shannon was 52 years old and in menopause. She had sleepwalking episodes as a child, but they diminished as she reached adolescence. Three months prior to her appointment, she was getting up and sleepwalking around the house. Her concerned husband gently guided her back to bed. He was worried she'd fall down the stairs. The incident became more regular, occurring three times a week. Usually, she went back to bed on her own, and sometimes she would lie down on the living room couch and continue sleeping until morning. Once in a while, Shannon's husband found her in a closet. She had no recollection of these events when he spoke to her about them but she believed him. She knew she was sleepwalking because she found herself waking up some mornings in another room.

Shannon felt pins and needles in her legs as she fell asleep. Sometimes these prevented her from falling asleep and other times they would wake her up in the middle of the night. In addition, her husband noted that her legs "keep moving all night even when she is fast asleep." After a sleep study, we determined that Shannon had a lot of periodic leg movements, about 50 to 60 an hour. About 20 of them were associated with mini-arousals that she was unaware of. She did not sleepwalk in our lab that night. However, her sleepwalking was becoming dangerous and more frequent. So I started her on a medication called pramipexole (Mirapex) that works for both restless legs syndrome and periodic limb movement disorder.

In the meantime I checked her ferritin, iron, and total iron capacity, and found that she did have low iron levels, causing her pins and needles symptoms of RLS. I placed her on iron in the form of ferrous sulfate tablets taken with vitamin C on an empty stomach three times a day. The latter improves the absorption of iron. Three months later, her iron levels were normal. When the deficiency was corrected, the RLS went away, as did her periodic limb movement. Her husband reported that she was no longer sleepwalking or moving as much in the middle of the night.

Night Terrors

NIGHT TERRORS IN CHILDREN

Night terrors typically occur in children between the ages of three and twelve years, with a peak onset in children aged three and one-half years old. An estimated 1% to 6% of children experience night terrors. Night terrors are not to be confused with nightmares or bad dreams. During a night terror, children may bolt upright, look fearful or panicked, and cry inconsolably. They may also sweat or thrash their limbs. Although children may seem to be awake during a night terror, they will be unresponsive to attempts to communicate with them, and may not recognize others familiar to them. The disorder usually resolves during adolescence.

If the episodes are recurring with a frequency of every night or three times a week, visit your pediatrician. Most likely, you'll receive a referral to a sleep center. Be prepared to share information about your child's sleep habits including:

- Does he or she snore?
- Complain of the legs itching, cramping, or feeling like pins and needles?
- Move restlessly in the night, especially moving his or her legs?

This information will help your doctor determine any precipitating factors that may be contributing to the night terrors, such as restless legs syndrome, and work with you to resolve them to eliminate the night terrors.

NIGHT TERRORS IN ADULTS

Night terrors are far less common for adults than sleepwalking, though patients frequently experience both night terrors and sleepwalking. Night terrors occur most often in people with post-traumatic stress disorder. As with children, night terrors in adults are characterized by sitting up, looking terrified, sweating, and perhaps screaming. The person may even run out of the house. They will not remember the event and usually it is the bed partner who is most terrified and prompts treatment.

Possible triggers include:

- High stress or anxiety
- Mental health issues
- Circadian issue, such as shiftwork
- Sleep apnea
- Periodic leg movement
- RLS
- Pharmaceutical factors (prescription and over-the-counter)

Adult night terrors often respond to treatments to rectify causes of poor quality or quantity of sleep. If testing reveals no cause, and the condition becomes frequent and potentially dangerous, then clonazepam is recommended. The antidepressant paroxetine may also be effective.

Answers to Your Questions

LITHIUM AND SLEEPWALKING

Q. I was diagnosed with bipolar disorder a year ago and was put on lithium. I have done very well on it. I live alone and frequently find myself waking up in a room other than my bedroom. Could this be because of the medication? I did not do this before.

A. Yes. Although lithium is an excellent medication, there is an increased incidence of sleepwalking noted in those who take it. I would bring this up with your prescribing health care provider. You may need to be switched to a different medication.

SLEEPWALKING AND GENETICS

Q. Is it true that sleepwalking is hereditary? My dad was a sleepwalker and now my son is sleepwalking.

A. Yes, many studies show genetics are involved in sleep-walking. We think that heredity may predispose one to sleepwalking, but there are other factors such as lack of sleep or a sleep disorder such as sleep apnea that may precipitate them.

DRIVING IN SLEEP?

Q. Can people drive in their sleep?

A. Yes they can. In fact it has been reported in Ambien users more often than with any other sleep aid. However, it can occur even in the absence of medications. It is a form of sleepwalking called sleep driving. There is a dissociation of the higher cortical brain centers from the motor centers in the brainstem.

ADULT SLEEPWALKING?

Q. My wife is 33 years old. She sleepwalks several times a week. This has been going on for several years. Isn't this supposed to be a disorder of children? Is there anything I should do?

A. Interestingly, 2% of adults sleepwalk. Less than 1% of these adult sleepwalkers do it frequently. If they do, as in your wife's case, there may be one of several contributing factors. First of all, is she getting enough sleep? Sleep deprivation can be a leading cause of sleepwalking. Is she under undue stress? This can also contribute to frequent sleepwalking. Finally, does she snore or have to get up in the middle of the night because her legs bother her? Sleep apnea and RLS are major contributors to sleepwalking in adults. With appropriate treatment, in most cases the sleepwalking goes away. I would recommend you discuss this matter with your health care professional.

9

Sexsomnia

Nothing is improbable until it moves into past tense.
—GEORGE ADE

Some bed partners might be thrilled when one initiates fondling and snuggling. If you are the partner on the receiving end, however, you could find it disconcerting when you realize your partner is asleep. Sex while sleeping? Is it possible?

Lew, aged 52, fondled and kissed his wife Kris, and then attempted intercourse . . . all in his sleep. This sudden behavior after 15 years of marriage was surprising to Kris, and even offensive when she realized he did not remember the episode the next morning. When she woke him during the event, he remembered nothing. Lew had never done this before.

Stories like Lew's describe a sleeping disorder called sleep sex, which causes people to act out sexual behaviors during sleep. Dr. Colin Shapiro named this sleep disorder sexsomnia in 2003, but reports have been rare to date. Two doctors, Schenck and Mahowald, published the outcomes of 31 cases found as a result of their survey of medical literature. This brought the topic of sleep sex out of the closet and to the attention of both medical doctors as well as the public through popular news articles.

One specific case presented in the book *Case Studies in Sleep Neurology: Common and Uncommon Presentations* shows how different or bizarre these nocturnal events seem if you experience them without further understanding or help. In this case, a married couple of 10 years went to a sleep disorders clinic to discuss the wife's nighttime behavior. The wife reported sleepwalking as a child that almost abated in her teen years, then occurred once or twice in a decade. But after the onset of hepatitis, she had regular episodes of night behaviors that included waking in a restless condition and scolding her husband. These verbal harangues could last as long as an hour. On other occasions, she sleepwalked aimlessly, moved furniture around, and initiated sexual intercourse. Though her daytime personality was that of a respectful, kind woman, and she didn't remember the behaviors, she did believe her husband's accounts of the events.

Can you imagine their sleepless nights? Can you feel the husband's fear grip his gut, knowing any verbal assault could expand into a long, irate monologue on yet another night?

You probably have not heard of sexsomnia because those who experience sleep sex are too embarrassed to discuss odd sex behaviors with a family physician. Yet, sexsomnia events occur nightly, and those who experience them suffer from fear, fatigue, unclear thinking, and low-grade chronic stress. Are you one of these people? Will you get help?

Sexsomnia Behaviors

The American Academy of Sleep Medicine officially recognized sexsomnia as a sleep disorder in 2005, and later the International Classification of Sleep Disorders also listed sleep sex as a disorder. Like sleepwalking and night terrors, sexsomnia is a parasomnia, an undesirable complex behavior associated with or arising from sleep that occurs during non-rapid eye movement (non-REM) sleep. The higher brain centers, such as the frontal lobes and prefrontal cortex, remain in a sleep state but the brain stem, which governs motor movement for basic functions like walking, eating, and sexual activity, remains active. The limbic system—the brain structures for emotion, emotional memory, gratification, and motivation—are wildly alive during sexsomnia episodes.

The official list of sexsomnia behaviors includes:

- Sexual talk and vocalizations, like moaning or groaning
- Body movements such as oral sex, thrusting against or penetrating the anus or vagina, and full intercourse
- Sexual touching like fondling, masturbating one's self or another

Another sexsomnia symptom is no memory of the events when awake. The amnesia factor makes sexsomnia the fodder for popular media stories of defense tactics in criminal cases of alleged sexual crimes like assault and rape. A popular media story might go like this:

Jake is a young, single man who drops by a regular Friday night party at his coworker's house. TGIF permeates the drinking mood. The music grows louder and new, unfamiliar faces replace those of coworkers. Jake makes new friends, engaging in conversation and dancing until fatigue and alcohol catch up to him. He crashes on his friend's couch just as he has on other Friday nights. An unfamiliar female sits down on the couch, closes her eyes, rests her head on the back of the couch to relax, and falls asleep. In the early morning hours, the woman jerks Jake out of a deep sleep, accusing him of fondling her.

She yells, "What are you doing? Why are touching me?"

Jake doesn't know and was not aware of the activity. In fact, Jake was just as surprised as the woman.

If the woman had not awakened and accused Jake of the inappropriate touching, he would have never known he was capable of such an act.

Causes

If one of your parents or grandparents walked while asleep, you may also. Researchers have shown a genetic link. Other common causes in my patients are sleep apnea, restless legs syndrome, or periodic limb movement that could cause arousal out of deep sleep. Once we treated the primary disorder, the trigger, the sexsomnia went away.

Other possible causes include medications such as Ambien, antidepressants, seizure-related drugs, recreational drugs, excessive consumption of alcohol, unusual stressors, post-traumatic stress, and REM behavioral disorder—a parasomnia that occurs out of dream sleep and can manifest itself as sexual behavior.

Are There Solutions?

If you feel you are experiencing symptoms, consult with a sleep expert. At your consultation, they will most likely ask you for:

- A thorough review of all medical records.
- A review of your lifestyle, stressors, sleep habits, and medications. Be sure to relate in complete honesty any of these: episodes of panic or anxiety, alcohol consumption levels, regularity of drinking, drug use including prescription and nonprescription medications.

- A sleep history of your family by blood—to help in determining a genetic component.
- An independent, detailed description of the sleep sex behaviors before the incident and behavior immediately after—checking here for confusion, dream mentation, arousal stupor, or amnesia.
- If violent behaviors have occurred, details about when, how often, level of violence, and the results.
- Finally, you might expect a sleep study, which takes place in a comfortable sleep center. An associate will monitor your sleep for rhythms and regularities in brain waves, breathing, heartbeat, sleep cycles, and movement patterns.

Eliminating other sleep disorders that may be triggering sexsomnia is the highest priority. If the determined cause is stress-related, exercise, better sleep hygiene (including an appropriate sleep schedule), or activities such as yoga or meditation will help. Certain medications, such as clonazepam, a form of benzodiazepine used to treat panic and anxiety disorders, can help to alleviate symptoms.

Importance of Getting Help

Bella shared that her husband Geoffrey, who masturbates while asleep, is not aware of his behavior while doing it. He has no recollection the next morning when Bella tells him what happened. Bella called his name during these episodes, attempting to wake him. Geoffrey's eyes appeared glassy with a far-off gaze. While Bella is concerned about the behavior, Geoffrey is embarrassed and doesn't want to see a sleep doctor.

Geoffrey is not alone in his embarrassment or in his thinking that he cannot be helped. Some patients who find their way to me believe that this nocturnal behavior is peculiar to them, since it is not exactly a popular topic of party conversation. Patient education, leading to some form of acceptance and a treatment protocol, brings much needed relief to the sufferer of sexsomnia.

Before Bella and Geoffrey made an appointment at the sleep clinic, one of Geoffrey's episodes ended in violence. As he made sexual advances to Bella during sleep, she pushed him away from her and called his name. When he did not respond, she gripped his shoulders and shook him again, calling, "Geoffrey . . ." He pushed into her and his weight rolled her off of the bed. When her face hit the nightstand, her nose bled. The first thing she thought was, *would her cowork-ers question her bruises tomorrow?* "Did he hit you? That nice man? Are you going to report this? You guys never argue; what happened?" Geoffrey himself was mortified when he learned about it. The incident caused them to pick up the phone and make an appointment. Embarrassed or not, the time for help had arrived.

Recently, I have received more questions about abnormal sexual behavior associated with sleep from readers of my weekly newspaper column and my Internet blog, both titled *Answers for Sleep.* In one instance, the reader's daughter was concerned because her new husband was instigating sexual activity while asleep. In another, the bed partner and other family members in their bedrooms noted loud moaning that resembled vocalizations associated with sexual activity.

People react differently to sexsomnia incidents. Some couples take the events in stride, finding opportunity for bet-ter sex or deeper conversation. Others are embarrassed and concerned. The person behind the acts may end up feeling deeply ashamed and become depressed. In other instances, since most are unaware of their behavior, they feel as if their bed partner made up the story. Communication and trust erode easily when you're tired and on edge and wondering *what's wrong with me.*

The important point for couples that experience sleep sex is to bring the behaviors to the attention of your health care provider. A thorough medical history, with a complete sleep analysis, including an overnight sleep study called polysomnography, could reveal the cause. Most patients' conditions are treatable. A recent study from Stanford found that out of 11 patients, 10 were successfully treated and the sexsomnia was eliminated.

Unfortunately, if ignored, sexsomnia behavior may lead to physical harm to the bed partner. There have been incidents where the police were called and legal action taken. Violence has also occurred in cases where the bed partner or a family member attempted to wake the sleeping person.

Sexsomnia as a Defense

Serious sexual scenarios involving children or violence have played out in courtrooms where sleep sex is used as a defense.

Most recently, the first case in Denmark using a sexsomnia defense went to court. The defender of a 32-year-old man who was accused of sexually assaulting two 17-year-old girls in 2011, claimed and proved that the accused suffered from a sleep disorder that caused him to act out sexual behaviors while asleep. Previous girlfriends of the accused verified they experienced similar behaviors with the defendant. The court dismissed the case on the grounds that the defense proved their case.

In a 2005 Canadian case, the court acquitted a man of sexually assaulting a woman who awakened him after both fell asleep at the house where they attended a party. The accused admitted he had been drinking. All he could say about the sexual assault was that he had no memory of it. No memory implied there was no intent to commit the act. His defense also proved he had a medical condition, a sleep disorder, in which sexual behaviors were performed and, of course, witnessed by the accuser.

In similar prosecuted cases in the United States and in Britain, some of the accused were acquitted while other defendants were found guilty. The forensic evidence is summarized in the following paragraph, which explains the unconscious action, the amnesia that happens in sexsomnia. The term *somnambulism* refers to sleepwalking, and the term *automatism* refers to the unconscious nature or automatic, uncontrolled behavior of sleep sex.

> *Somnambulism or sleepwalking is a viable defence on the basis of automatism. The behaviours that occur during sleepwalking can be highly complex and include sexual behaviour of all types. Somnambulistic sexual behaviour (also called sexsomnia, sleep sex) is considered a variant of sleepwalking disorder as the overwhelming majority of people with sexsomnia have a history of parasomnia and a family history of sleepwalking.*

As I see it, the defense should consider the presence of obvious sleep disorders such as sleep apnea or another sleep disturbance to explain the cause of arousal from deep, delta-wave sleep, also known as slow-wave sleep. They should also consider sleepwalking, night terrors, epilepsy, or a REM sleep behavior disorder. Each of these could cause nocturnal sexual behaviors. The testimony by one or several additional witnesses, such as previous bed partners or family members, could verify previous sex sleep behavior. This is very important to show that sexual behavior while asleep is prominent in the history of the defendant, since sexsomnia is repetitive. The intention to commit the crime would be nonexistent in persons who have sexsomnia, because they have no memory of the event. Horrified and mortified that they could commit the act, they make no attempt to hide or lie about it. Such defendants are not normally evasive.

Answers to Your Questions

MEDICATIONS

Q. What medicines are used for sexsomnia?

A. The most commonly used medication is called clonazepam. This drug is also used in refractory sleepwalking. However, eliminating alcohol and looking for an underlying primary sleep disorder that might be triggering the episodes is paramount.

STRESS

Q. My live-in girlfriend complained of me trying to have sex with her in my sleep for the third time. I wake up with no recollection of doing anything and am worried for her safety. I had a couple episodes of sleepwalking when I was young, but no other history of actions during my sleep. I have noticed that each time I've had a "sexsomniac slip" she and I had gone to bed upset with each other. Could stress be causing me to do this? Is there any way to lessen my chances of doing things I don't want to without medication?

A. Yes, stress as well as sleep deprivation, medications, and primary sleep disorders such as sleep apnea, can be the cause. I think it is important that you consult with a sleep specialist in your area. A thorough sleep workup would seem to be indicated.

10

The Night Eaters

The bed is a bundle of paradoxes: we go to it with reluctance, yet we quit it with regret; we make up our minds every night to leave it early, but we make up our bodies every morning to keep it late.
—OGDEN NASH

Eating and sleeping are two of our most basic biological needs, both controlled by the natural circadian rhythm of our bodies. Normal processes include a delicate balance of chemistry—most notably between glucose, insulin, and the hormone leptin—that regulates appetite and metabolism while we sleep. When this rhythm is out of balance, disorders affecting our sleep and eating habits can result. A. J. Stunkard, a medical doctor who identified night eating syndrome and eventually founded the Center for Weight and Eating Disorders at the University of Pennsylvania's Perelman School of Medicine, found the underlying cause to be a misfiring of the circadian rhythm that resulted in delayed meal timing.

Sleep-related eating disorders are relatively rare, affecting only 1% to 5% of the population; however, they are severely disruptive to the person's physical and mental well-being, causing obesity and sometimes, other risky behaviors. They are also indicative of other underlying problems such as genetic predispositions, hormonal and neurochemical disturbances, and mood disorders. Individuals with an eating disorder also often have sleep disorders.

The Two Forms of Night Eating

In night eating disorders, the circadian eating cycle is out of phase with the circadian sleep–wake cycle. The sleep–wake cycle remains relatively normal, but the timing of eating is out of sync, resulting in over 30% of caloric intake to occur after dinner. There are two forms of night eating, and both disorders are characterized by the high intake of simple sugars and fats, causing weight gain. Both also occur during non–rapid eye movement (non-REM) sleep.

Sleep-related eating disorder is associated with disrupted sleep, weight gain, and major chronic morbidity. It is a type of sleepwalking with onset associated with several medications such as Ambien (zolpidem), as well as with other sleep disorders such as obstructive sleep apnea, periodic limb movement, and restless legs syndrome (RLS).

In this disorder, the night eater usually has total amnesia of the trips to the kitchen and eating. In fact, many of these people wake up with food in their bed or stove burners left on and no recollection of what happened.

Night eating syndrome, the second form, refers to the eater being conscious while engaged in uncontrollable eating after bedtime. It is not unusual for these people to consume over 50% of their daily caloric intake after bedtime.

Sleep-Related Eating Disorder (SRED)

A sleep-related eating disorder refers to the patient who gets out of bed while asleep and eats. Sometimes the sleeper eats bizarre food or combinations of foods. The biggest dangers are:

1. Environmental, as in leaving a gas flame or an electric burner on, burning foods if cooking, using knives, or breaking glassware—the options are as numerous as the dangerous objects in your kitchen.
2. Personal, as in the case of a sleeper ingesting poison, drinking dish detergent, cutting him- or herself with a knife, and such.

Over the years, I have treated several patients with SRED. In terms of parasomnias, SRED is closely related to sleepwalking, and the sleeper may begin with sleepwalking and then move on to sleep eating. When this happens, eating usually becomes the primary sleep disorder activity.

Those suffering from SRED are usually fully asleep when they get out of bed, go to the kitchen, and begin eating (although some have reported being "half-awake, half-asleep"). Research shows that for most patients, this occurs during slow-wave sleep, which is a deep, non-REM phase. They put on weight, are not hungry for breakfast in the morning, and report nonrestorative sleep and daytime fatigue. They eat large quantities of food that are high in carbohydrates, and these eating sessions are similar to bulimic binges. However, unlike bulimics, those with SRED do not purge. The more disturbing aspect of this condition is the possibility of eating the inedible or harmful substances, such as caustic acids. These episodes can occur on a nightly basis, and rarely more than once a night.

Often another person in the house is the first one to observe the clues to the disorder: food in the bed, a stove burner left on, a mess in the kitchen, or finding the sleeper engaged in the eating behavior. These episodes have been described as "involuntary" and "out of control," which can later be confirmed by monitoring the person in a sleep clinic. The sleep technician would report that the sleeper showed bodily movements like chewing or eating when food was left next to the bed. Of course, the person's lack of awareness presents an entirely different set of dangers such as self-injury.

SRED was first identified in 1991, and has recently received media attention because of an association with the sleep aid Ambien. Also known as zolpidem, this drug is widely acknowledged as a cause of SRED in some cases and is part of a larger problem that includes sleepwalking and sleep driving. For most people, SRED has an underlying sleep-related cause, such as obstructive sleep apnea, RLS, or periodic limb movement disorder. According to one survey, 50% of patients with SRED had RLS. SRED has also been linked with daytime anxiety and other psychological issues. In the case of SRED, discontinuing the offending medication or treating the primary sleep disorder can be curative.

We eventually determined an underlying sleep-related cause at the root of Janice's trouble. Janice, a 23-year-old woman, had been experiencing daytime fatigue for the past several months, even though her sleep habits had not changed. Despite going to bed at a reasonable hour each night and sleeping for eight hours, she never felt refreshed. She had not changed her eating habits either, but had gained several pounds, which distressed her. Janice came to the clinic after her partner, Jon, found her in the kitchen at 1:30 a.m. Jon observed that Janice had opened the refrigerator and had placed assorted foods like mustard, one bag of deli meat, a jar of dill pickles, and frozen ice cream bars on the kitchen counter, and she was eating a dill pickle with mustard. She also seemed to be asleep and didn't respond when Jon called her name, asking if anything was wrong.

The next day, Janice had no recollection of what had happened. Since then, Jon observed the same behavior three more times and became alarmed when he saw her pouring cleaning fluid into a drinking glass. He led her back to bed before she could drink it.

I could see Janice was relieved to be getting help for her "bizarre" story, as she described it. Upon waking in the morning, she had no recollection of eating anything or even getting out of bed. I advised Janice and her partner Jon to remove all knives and other sharp objects, as well as any dangerous chemicals, from the kitchen before bedtime. She told me she had a history of occasional sleepwalking over the years. She also related that her mother had been known to sleepwalk.

After taking her history, I arranged a sleep study for Janice. She would spend a night in the sleep clinic, as this appeared to be a classic case of sleep eating. The reason for doing a sleep study was that we were looking for an underlying sleep disorder that might be triggering these undesirable behaviors.

In couples like Janice and John, I have to be very matter of fact. As time goes on, they may become lax in keeping to the specific instructions I give them. Removing the toxic or dangerous materials from the kitchen is not a choice. It must be done. Jon needs an alarm sensor or bed pad sensor so he wakes up when Janice gets out of bed and can gently guide her back to bed to prevent her from harming or even killing herself.

The results of Janice's sleep study through polysomnography revealed that Janice exhibited numerous arousals from sleep during the night, all while in a deep or slow-wave sleep phase. This was important because most SRED occurs out of this stage of sleep. We determined that Janice had sleep apnea that was causing these arousals. We started her on continuous positive airway pressure (CPAP) titration to treat the sleep apnea and within a few weeks Janice's symptoms began to improve; her bingeing sessions became less frequent over time, and she felt more rested during the day. She also began losing weight. It's been over a year and Janice has had no more episodes of SRED.

TREATMENT OPTIONS

First, it is essential to resolve any underlying sleep problems that could be triggering the SRED. Pharmacological treatments for SRED include clonazepam, a benzodiazepine commonly used for uncontrolled sleepwalkers; pramipexole, an agent that stimulates dopamine receptors in the nervous system and is used frequently for RLS; and topiramate, an antiseizure medication that has been found to have appetite-suppressing ability. While many patients have reported success with these treatments, there are no guarantees. I still advise patients to make their living environment as safe as possible.

Night Eating Syndrome (NES)

Twenty-five-year-old Susan had been suffering from anorexia since she was a teenager. Over several years of psychotherapy treatment, she was able to maintain a healthy weight. However, her diet was still regimented and controlled. She also suffered from occasional bouts of depression. In recent months, Susan woke often in the middle of the night with a strong desire to eat. She did not recall feeling particularly hungry, just a feeling that she would not be able to get back to sleep unless she ate. After trying unsuccessfully to resist, she would eventually go to the kitchen, where she consumed large quantities of food, and eventually gained weight with the intake. She consumed most of her calories after dinner, and arose from bed repeatedly to go to the kitchen.

I treated her with sertraline, which regulated her serotonin levels and helped her stay asleep throughout the night. She mentioned that her symptoms came and went, usually growing worse during more stressful periods. I recommended that Susan continue psychotherapy so that she could manage stress more effectively.

Susan's symptoms are associated with another sleep-related eating disorder called night eating syndrome (NES). In NES the biological clock for eating, the circadian eating cycle, is out of phase with the circadian sleep–wake cycle. The sleep–wake cycle remains relatively normal, but the timing of eating is out of sync and results in an average of over 30% of caloric intake occurring after dinner. This has been verified by studies showing the secretion of hormones that suppress appetite being released at atypical times with regards to the 24-hour day.

While it is similar to SRED, this disorder is associated with

- Daytime eating disorders, such as anorexia nervosa and bulimia
- Hormonal and chemical imbalances
- Mood disorders, such as bipolar

Those with NES often report evening hyperphagia—or an insatiable need to consume large quantities of food, which results in a lack of appetite for breakfast (morning anorexia). Between 30% and 50% of their daily caloric intake occurs after dinner, and they experience at least two of these nocturnal eating sessions a week. However, unlike SRED, NES does not usually involve ingesting inedible or dangerous substances.

Criteria for diagnosing NES were not formalized until 2008, during the First International Night Eating Symposium. Caloric intake and two nocturnal eating sessions are considered to be the first indicators of NES. For a definitive diagnosis the person must also have at least three of the following symptoms.

SYMPTOMS

1. Lack of desire to eat in the morning or breakfast is omitted at least four times per week.
2. A strong urge to eat after dinner and before going to bed. This desire may appear when the person wakes during the night.
3. Insomnia at least four nights a week (the person either has trouble falling asleep or staying asleep).
4. Must eat in order to fall or go back to sleep.
5. Experience frequent depression or a worsening of mood toward the latter part of the day.
6. The symptoms last at least three months.
7. The symptoms cause significant interference with the person's life.

A primary diagnosis of NES means that the symptoms are not secondary to substance abuse or dependence, medical disorders, medication, or other psychiatric disorders.

There is evidence that NES is genetic and is usually a chronic condition characterized by early adult onset. Over the years the symptoms may wane, then flare up again when the person is under stress.

In addition to eating disorders, NES has been associated with depression, substance abuse, and anxiety. It also makes it difficult for a person to maintain a healthy weight or lose weight. It is especially dangerous for those trying to manage diabetes. Given NES's co-morbidity with other problems, I often recommend that the patient undergo psychotherapy and phototherapy (light therapy) to improve mood.

NES can be treated in some cases with effective antidepressants, such as sertraline (Zoloft), which raise serotonin levels. Two other treatments include cognitive behavioral therapy and properly timed light therapy. In the latter, a light box emits light at various levels of intensity, measured in lux, which is the amount of light a patient gets when sitting at specified distances from the light box. You would use a light box every day for the duration and intensity the doctor suggests. For instance, if starting with 15 minutes each day for several days, the duration increases to the amount of time discussed with the sleep doctor. Cognitive behavioral therapy was first used to treat the thoughts associated with the need to eat because researchers learned the following thought distinguished NES from SRED: *If I don't eat, I won't be able to fall asleep.* A behavioral therapy approach to weight loss is effective, as is progressive relaxation.

Distinguishing SRED and NES

While SRED and NES are outwardly similar, there are a few other important distinctions.

Another way to differentiate the two is to think of SRED as primarily a sleep disorder that involves eating and NES as primarily an eating disorder that involves sleeping. In fact, the lack of research in this area is largely due to two groups of researchers—those who specialize in sleep disorders and those whose focus on eating disorders. The International Classification of Sleep Disorders has recently been revised to do away with the distinction. This may result in more thorough data collection because researchers will have a common objective.

Sleep-Related Eating Disorder	Night Eating Disorder
Non-REM slow-wave sleep	Non-REM sleep or awake
Associated with restless legs syndrome and sleep apneas	Associated with daytime eating disorders
Asleep during eating event, and recall of event could be partial to full amnesia	Fully awake when moving from bed to kitchen and remember incident
Involuntary eating in middle of night	Not typically a physical sensation of hunger
	Overeat between the evening meal and bedtime
	Feel they must eat in order to return to sleep
Unusual foodstuff, could be harmful	Eat more normal foods
Daytime fatigue	History of difficulty falling asleep or staying asleep throughout night (insomnia)
Mood changes Depression common	Mood disorders more frequent

Answers to Your Questions

WIFE EATS SUGAR

Q. At least three times a week, my wife goes to the kitchen during the night and eats. She has no recollection of doing this. When I awaken I often find open packages of sugar and candy on the counter. This seems to have started at about the same time she started a medication called Zyprexa for bipolar disorder. Do you think there could be a relationship?

A. Yes, Zyprexa (olanzapine) is one of several medications that have been associated with SRED. This is an abnormal behavior arising out of sleep, referred to as a parasomnia. It is very similar to sleepwalking in that the higher brain centers of the cortex are in a state of sleep while the brain stem is active. That is why there is frequently a complete amnesia for the event. Other medications that have been associated with this include Ambien (zolpidem), Halcion (triazolam), and lithium, as well as several other prescriptions for sleep medications and antipsychotics. I would definitely bring this to the attention of you health care provider.

ZOLPIDEM

Q. I have been having some problems with sleeping. Recently my doctor put me on a medication called zolpidem. It has done wonders for my sleep. However, about once a week I find that I have been eating in my sleep. I have no recollection of this. Could this be due to the medication?

A. Yes, quite likely. Zolpidem is the generic form of Ambien. Although an excellent sleep aid, an unfortunate side effect is SRED. In this disorder, people eat while they are actually asleep. It is a form of sleepwalking. I would bring this to the attention of your health care provider immediately. You will probably need to stop the medication.

WHAT CAN BE DONE?

Q. What can be done about eating during the night while half-asleep?

A. The key is whether you are actually asleep and have little or no recollection of going to the kitchen and eating, or are you awake but groggy when you are eating? The former is called SRED and is similar to sleepwalking. This can be caused by medications such as Ambien (zolpidem), as well as primary sleep disorders such as sleep apnea and RLS. Eliminating the offending medications or treating the underlying sleep disorder can treat this.

If you are unsure, I urge you to see a sleep specialist to work this out.

I AM AWAKE WHEN EATING AT NIGHT

Q. I have read about a disorder where people eat in the middle of the night. They say its like sleepwalking. I do most of my eating after bedtime, but I am awake. Is that the same thing?

A. No, what you are describing is called NES. In this disorder people consume over 25% of their daily calories after 6:00 p.m. However, unlike SRED, which is done while sleeping, they are wide awake and conscious of what they are doing. The two are not synonymous. In your case you are describing NES. There are several behavioral and pharmacological treatments for this condition. In fact, several of the antidepressants that increase serotonin levels such as sertraline (Zoloft) and citalopram (Celexa) have been found to be particularly effective.

Self-Check: Do You Have a Night Eating Disorder?

Repeatedly eating and drinking during the main sleep period, plus one or more of the following:

- Eating strange combinations of food or even inedible things
- Complaints of nonrestorative sleep, daytime fatigue, or somnolence
- Sleep-related injury
- Other risky behavior while looking for or making food
- Lack of appetite in the morning—morning anorexia
- Physical consequences of repeatedly bingeing (weight gain)
- Cannot be better explained by another sleep, medical, or eating disorder

11

Do You Sleep, but Not Too Deeply? REM Sleep Behavior Disorder

I'm not asleep . . . but that doesn't mean I'm awake.
—UNKNOWN

Recently, an interviewer asked me, "Is there one patient who has inspired you?" The patient who came to mind actually fascinated me and was one reason I became interested in sleep medicine. Early in the year 2000, I was just moving into the field of sleep science when a very pleasant woman arrived for an appointment. By the time she consulted with me, she had been to the local emergency room on several occasions. She had jumped out of her bed, onto the bedroom floor, and in every instance she was dreaming that she was diving into a pool. She had to receive stitches to repair the damage on each occasion. I arranged for her sleep study and we were able to document that she had significant and repetitive movements associated with rapid eye movement (REM) or dream sleep.

After hearing this patient's story, one of my goals became to shed more light on this problem. First, I had to learn about it myself. I started researching and quickly realized that she had a sleep disorder called REM sleep behavior disorder (RSBD), a disruption of normal REM sleep. During the REM phase of sleep, the part of the brain that makes the body still and unmoving allows your neurobiology to repair and restore. In RSBD, the brain does not receive the signal to be still and the patient is able to act out his or her dreams. Through the years since I've become an expert on this topic, I have learned that people with RSBD are able to physically act out their dreams, which can range from simple mumbling or other vocalizations to violent punching. Obviously, the violent action that could hurt a bed partner motivates people to see a sleep doctor.

When my patient returned, I told her the diagnosis and that she didn't need to be embarrassed. She was definitely relieved that she wasn't crazy, to use her words. The movement in her sleep had to do with some abnormalities of the circuitry that goes on between the brain stem and spinal cord. I prescribed a medication called clonazepam. This medication acts as a mild sedative and muscle relaxant for the sleeper with active limbs.

This patient saw me regularly for a couple of months, and one day she arrived practically in tears and announced, "Gosh, I'm not doing it anymore, Dr. Rosenberg!" We could not quit smiling because we shared the incredible feelings of the problem solved. No more trips to the ER because she had once again cracked her head on the floor after diving in her sleep.

This patient spurred me on to learn, since no one in our area of Lake Havasu, with the exception of a few physicians in Phoenix, knew anything about RSBD. That's the reason why that patient stands out for me. She was like my bridge from being only a sleep apnea doctor to a sleep specialist whose practice encompasses much more than treatment for apnea.

Symptoms

In the late 1980s, a group of researchers reported patients that were exhibiting signs of a new form of parasomnia, an umbrella term for a collection of strange sleep behaviors. Behaviors such as sleepwalking or sleep eating were studied previously and were found to occur during the non-REM stages of sleep. However, these new cases were different because they occurred during REM sleep. In addition to the normal eye movements for REM sleep, these patients vocalized sounds and had a notable *lack* of the atonia, the muscle paralysis, usually present in REM sleep. This was the first diagnosis of REM sleep behavioral disorder. We now know it is present in about one out of every 200 people. RSBD usually strikes around the age of 50, and mostly in men, whose wild and often violent dreams contradict their peaceful waking lives. The number of women being diagnosed with RSBD has recently been on the rise; however, their symptoms are usually milder.

Symptoms for RSBD include:

SYMPTOM CHECKLIST

1. "Motor attacks" ranging from simple movements such as twitches, jerks, and grimace, to complex behaviors such as searching movements, defensive and or aggressive actions, and vocal sounds. These behaviors are reactions to events occurring in the sufferers' vivid dreams.
2. Occurrence at least 90 minutes after sleep onset, but most oftentake place much later when REM sleep increases in duration.
3. Violent episodes typically happen about once per week but may appear as frequently as four times per night over several consecutive nights.
4. An acute, transient form may accompany REM rebound during withdrawal from alcohol and sedative-hypnotic

agents. Drug-induced cases have been reported with several antidepressants.

The Importance of Rapid Eye Movement (REM) Sleep

Chapter 2 provides a detailed description of a sleep cycle moving from non-REM stages to REM sleep or dream sleep, and how the sleep cycles repeat throughout your sleeping hours. REM refers to rapid eye movement and accounts for 20% to 25% of sleep time. If you were a sleep technician in a sleep lab, you would observe REM sleep as the sleeper's quickened eye movements and the EEG (electroencephalography) patterns of higher-frequency waves that rise and drop rapidly, a pattern referred to as the sawtooth wave. REM, the final stage of the sleep cycle, is also the lightest stage of sleep. The eye movement mimics that of the waking state, as well as brain activity equivalent to that of "relaxed wakefulness." We can dream during REM sleep.

Another feature distinguishing REM from other sleep stages is the paralysis of the body, called atonia, which serves to keep the sleeper still and receive positive, regenerative benefits that transpire. The amount of REM sleep we get depends largely on our age. REM comprises nearly 80% of sleep time in newborn babies, and then progressively decreases until it reaches 20% to 25%, which is normal for adults. Most people, if they are getting enough sleep, experience three to five periods of REM sleep per night, with each REM stage getting longer as the night progresses.

REM BENEFITS

Researchers have correlated REM sleep to abilities such as creativity and better problem-solving. We have found that the term "sleep on it" works because in a REM state, the brain makes connections among one's daily experiences and correlates them to experiences or past memories. However, the quality of sleep matters more than the duration of sleep. Sleep experts agree that REM sleep has a "global effect on the physiological processes regulated by the brain" and performs numerous housekeeping functions. One function is to process the day's memories, particularly those involving emotions and stress, through a complex, chemical process that controls neurons in several areas of the brain.

REM sleep is critical to learning and retaining information, such as language or how-to skills such as playing a piano. It also helps with cognitive development in infants and children, which may explain why they get so much more REM sleep than adults. This is also connected to the earlier theory about dreaming, which was illustrated in a 2001 study conducted by MIT professor Matt Wilson.

In the first stage of the experiment, Wilson implanted multiple electrodes into the brains of his lab rats. Then he trained them to run through mazes, measuring the activity of the neurons in the hippocampus. After determining that each maze created a unique pattern of neural activity, Wilson measured the rats' brain activity again, this time while they were sleeping. Wilson was amazed by the results of his 45 recorded rat dreams, 20 of which were exact replicas of the mazes they ran during the first phase. The rats were using the REM sleep period to consolidate their memories and learn new things. Now imagine all the new skills an infant learns each day. No wonder they need so much REM sleep!

Other studies show that for REM sleep to be useful in integrating learning, an emotional component to the information is required for being consolidated or memorized. Neutral information is better processed during a different part of the sleep cycle. There is much evidence of this theory among many famous artists, writers, and scientists, who have found inspiration in their dreams. Musicians from Billy Joel and Paul McCartney to Beethoven have stated that they first heard a song in their dreams, and writers Edgar Allan Poe and Mary Shelley often dreamed their story ideas.

Furthermore, through dream symbols and metaphors, scientists have found solutions to complex problems they could not uncover while awake. German chemist August Kekulé went to bed one night, frustrated with his lack of success on his latest project. Kekulé dreamed about two snakes whose tails and mouths met to form circles, and upon awakening he realized that the structure of the compound he searched for was not a straight line but a circular one. This is even more incredible when one realizes that, at the time, all known organic compounds were linear. Thanks to his dream, Kekulé went down in history as the man who discovered the benzene molecule. Others have also achieved success after awaking from REM sleep. Inventor Elias Howe's dream aided him in inventing the sewing machine, and Jack Nicklaus improved his golf game after he found himself holding his club differently—in a dream.

Are you wondering why you haven't had some magical dream that led you to a groundbreaking discovery? The answer may lie in the above examples. These people were dreaming about things they were very passionate about in their waking lives. This passion may have sparked the revelations in REM sleep.

Clearly, there are many benefits of REM sleep—it helps us integrate, consolidate, and learn information we've collected throughout the day. Through REM sleep, we process our emotions. Studies also show that when people don't get enough REM sleep their bodies play catch-up or get "rebound" REM sleep.

LACK OF REM SLEEP

When REM sleep is missing or interrupted, people lose the opportunity to process the emotional events of their day. This explains why those suffering from disorders that interrupt REM sleep, such as obstructive or central sleep apnea, often develop secondary disorders such as anxiety, obsessive–compulsive disorder (OCD), and post-traumatic stress disorder (PTSD). (For more information on this, please see chapter 7 on apneas or chapter 12 on PTSD.)

When one considers the short amount of time spent in REM sleep, as opposed to non-REM sleep or waking, the effects of REM sleep deficiency show how critical REM is for mental and physical well-being. A lack of REM sleep affects nearly every physiological process, most notably in persons with clinical depression. Lack of REM sleep can also impair memory and inhibit certain kinds of learning.

Less REM sleep means more non-REM sleep when norepinephrine and serotonin levels are higher, but not as high as during wakefulness. People who are deficient in REM sleep are more reactive to stimuli than normal. However, lack of REM sleep does not make one overreact to a stimulus that normally does not affect them.

New evidence establishes RSBD as a predictor of neurological diseases such as Parkinson's, Lewy body dementia, and others. Thirty to forty percent of those with RSBD are diagnosed with a neurological disease. A team at the Mayo Clinic (Rochester, MN) analyzed the brain autopsy findings from 172 patients with a RSBD, of which 83% were men. The mean age was 62 years for the RSBD onset, and the diagnosis preceded Parkinson's by a mean of 6 years in 151 patients. The diagnosis preceded death by an average of 13 years.

Treatment Options

Patients come to the sleep clinic to explore the acting out of dreams, such as leaping, diving, and running, usually in bed and sometimes violently, during REM sleep. The acting out behavior can be directed toward a partner, and the patient can also wake up or be awakened.

The best way for a sleep specialist to diagnose RSBD is the use of video polysomnography, where the sleeping person is recorded for a full night's sleep. The sleep specialist evaluates the study to see if there is increased paradoxical movement during REM sleep. The sleep specialist determines if there are other disorders such as sleepwalking, seizures, or agitated arousal out of REM sleep due to sleep apnea that could explain the abnormal behaviors. If a patient or family member complains of violent behaviors during sleep that is associated with dreaming, we are looking for increasing muscle movement in REM sleep. That confirms it.

If needed, the sleep specialist will collect information through clinical interviews as well as screening questionnaires regarding the person's sleep history. The patient's sleep partner will verify the answers concerning:

- The frequency of the motor attacks or behaviors
- The amount of time between the events or attacks
- How long they last

When a diagnosis of RSBD has been made, your treatment may include:

- Physical safeguards to prevent injury: These may include adding pads to your floor or barriers to your bed. For example, one man in his sixties had a tendency to be so active that he often threw himself out of bed while asleep. A simple harness-type halter around his chest and connected to the bedpost kept him from violent injuries.

- Medications: A tranquilizer of the benzodiazepine class such as clonazepam, is usually prescribed. Recently, melatonin has been found to be very effective.

Answers to Your Questions

FIGHTING FOR HIS LIFE

Q. My husband has violent dreams. Over the last few months, he has begun flailing and screaming in his sleep. If I awaken him, he says he was fighting for his life. This started about the time he was placed on an antidepressant. Could this be the cause?

A. Yes, it is quite possible. What you are describing is called RSBD. It is the loss of the normal state of paralysis during dream (REM) sleep that occurs in most us. It has been associated with many neurodegenerative diseases. However, it is also seen in association with some antidepressants. Several antidepressants including paroxetine, fluoxetine, imipramine, and venlafaxine, as well as some blood pressure medications called beta-blockers have occasionally been implicated. I would bring this to the attention of your health care provider at once.

MEDICATION FOR REM SLEEP BEHAVIOR DISORDER (RSBD)

Q. My husband has been acting out his dreams for several years and I have been injured several times. Consequently, I now sleep in a separate bed. He had a sleep test that confirmed that he has a disorder called RSBD. His doctor, on the advice of the sleep specialist who read his sleep study, placed him on a medication called clonazepam. Unfortunately, it has not worked. We have since moved to another state. Any ideas? Is there anything else that might work?

A. I would suggest that you seek out a board-certified specialist in sleep disorders as they are familiar with the latest therapies. Several studies have shown success in treating this disorder with melatonin and also a drug called pramipexole, the latter commonly used in Parkinson's disease. There are anecdotal reports of other medications that are effective, but the aforementioned are the best alternatives. Additionally, it is important to make sure that he is not taking any medications that can cause or exacerbate the condition. In several of my patients and in the sleep literature, discontinuation of these medications can result in an improved response to medical treatment.

ACTING OUT IN DREAMS

Q. I have a habit of acting out my dreams. I've been doing this for many years. In fact, my wife sleeps in another room rather than risk injury. I saw a sleep specialist and he told me I'd have to have an overnight sleep study to make a diagnosis. My question is, why do I need a test? Isn't it obvious what I am doing?

A. Unfortunately, these things are not that clear-cut. The specialist thinks you have a disorder called RSBD. This is a condition characterized by the ability to move during dream sleep (REM). It is present in about one out of 200 people. Unfortunately, there are other sleep disorders such as sleepwalking and seizures that can look just like this disorder. That is why it is necessary for you to be studied in a sleep lab. The therapies for these various disorders are by no means the same.

SCREAMING AND THRASHING

Q. My 60-year-old husband has been acting strangely in his sleep. Several times a week he starts screaming and thrashing about in his sleep. On several occasions, I have had to get out of bed to avoid being struck by him. He tells me he was dreaming. This is frightening me, as I am worried he will hurt himself or me. I spoke to my health care provider who suggested my husband see a psychiatrist. What could be going on here?

A. It sounds as if your husband is suffering from RSBD. This is a condition where people are able to move during dream sleep. Normally, when we enter dream sleep, also known as REM sleep, we become paralyzed. That protects us and those around us from our acting out of our dreams. This disorder is more common in older men and is treatable. I recommend you have him see a sleep medicine specialist.

I MOVED TO A DIFFERENT BEDROOM

Q. My husband is 52 years old. During the last year, he has become violent while sleeping. He kicks and punches. This happens about four times a month. I have had to move into a separate bedroom. A friend tells me her husband was doing this and he was placed on a medication called clonazepam. Should I request that my health care provider put my husband on this medication?

A. No, not yet. Your husband is evidencing what we call VBS— violent behavior associated with sleep. There are numerous causes such as sleepwalking, RSBD (a disorder of dream enactment), and nocturnal seizures, to name a few. It is very important that your husband undergoes a thorough sleep evaluation, including a sleep study. That should pinpoint the cause and result in appropriate treatment.

WATCHPAT DEVICE

Q. Recently, I saw a doctor about my insomnia since I have trouble staying asleep. Sometimes I have vivid dreams and actually act them out. He suggested that I get a sleep study at home. He has a new device they call a WatchPAT. Can you tell me about it?

A. The WatchPAT and other portable home devices are good only for diagnosing sleep apnea. They monitor arterial tone, body movement, and drops in oxygen. Unfortunately, they are useless in diagnosing myriad other sleep-related conditions. These devices are unable to detect in what stage of sleep you are. They cannot detect problems such as periodic limb movement disorder, which frequently accompanies restless legs syndrome, or adverse medication effects on sleep. In your case, it sounds as if you may have REM behavior disorder. This condition results in abnormal movement during dream sleep. I recommend that you discuss with your health care provider a fully attended diagnostic sleep study in a sleep lab.

REM SLEEP ABNORMALITY?

Q. Recently, my wife underwent a sleep study because of her chronic insomnia. She wakes up frequently throughout the night and does not know why. During the test, they noted that she moved a lot while in dream sleep. Her doctor said this could be due to a sleep abnormality called RSBD. I looked this up and it says these people act out their dreams. We have been married for over 30 years and I can definitely say she does not. What do you think?

A. Increased movement during dream sleep is needed to make a diagnosis of RSBD. However, it also requires a history of dream-enacting behavior. Without that, one cannot call it RSBD. Still, about 25% of people that present with this finding in a sleep lab will go on to develop the full-blown disorder.

PART FOUR

Sleep Disorders and Major Health Issues

Sleep disorders coexist with other medical problems that disrupt sleep, such as post-traumatic stress disorder (PTSD) and attention deficit hyperactivity disorder (ADHD). It is essential to treat both issues.

12

Sleep for Those with Post-Traumatic Stress Disorder

The pain and the memories will never go away. I wish I could sleep one night without nightmares.

—PATIENT WITH PTSD

Could sound, long sleep be a health solution for those diagnosed with post-traumatic stress disorder (PTSD)? In short, yes. Recent studies reveal that treatment focusing on sleep alleviates both sleep disturbances and the severity of PTSD symptoms.

Gina's Story

Gina attended a private high school in an Atlanta suburb and was approaching her sixteenth birthday in the middle of a very active junior year. She stayed after school for a cheerleading meeting with the squad's sponsor to plan for the next semester after Christmas break. She entered the bathroom before heading to the meeting. Two high school boys in the empty hallway followed her into the bathroom. They attacked her from the back and threw her to the floor; they pinned her down, slapped her around, and raped her several times.

Gina and her parents reported the incident to the school and the police. The boys were charged, and a trial date would be set eventually.

Meantime, Gina withdrew from her social activities and could not muster the courage to return to classes at the high school. Rather, she focused her time and attention on accelerated high school courses for the gifted via an online portal. Her gifted mind kept her busy in exploring, learning, and creating, but the rape was not distant. She relived the experiences but she never told her parents. She appeared to be studying and working hard, but she had to force her effort, and sometimes do the same task several times, like trying to see through fog.

Her resilience amazed me as I came to know Gina better during her first appointment at the sleep disorders clinic to discuss her medical history.

"Welcome, Gina. I'm so glad that you decided to explore getting more help. Your therapist indicated she thought your sleeping issues should be addressed before continuing in more depth with her. I understand the trauma you went through from your therapist's input and medical records. Can you tell me more about what you have been experiencing?"

"Yes, I can, and thank you for seeing me. I know I need help, and I try to control everything that comes up with me so my parents don't freak out any more than they already do. My new therapist is great, but she says I need more help from you, and she gave me some tools to get started. First of all, I am having nightmares, like replays of the rape. The memories seem to creep in when they want to, not like they have a schedule, and usually it is at night. My therapist said the experience could come any time, day or night, but . . ."

"Gina, does that happen every night? Or maybe several times a week?"

"Oh! Thanks for reminding me. My therapist said to keep a journal, like a log." Gina pulled out a spiral-bound journal with attractive pink roses. She caught me looking at the roses.

"Pretty, aren't they? They make me smile, so I sketch roses and doodle flowers." She laughed as she explained to me that her doodling was her art therapy, and then opened the journal, and reported that within the last 14 days, she had nightmares 10 times. The nightmares were not always long dream episodes.

"Dr. Rosenberg, there are a few other things going on. Some nights, I cannot go to sleep at all. If I am exhausted and sleep a little when my head hits the pillow, it feels like I am still awake and going through the nightmare. I try to be cheerful around my parents, but I feel like I am sinking into a hole. Sometimes at night I get headaches, and just crying seems to help when a headache hits. Other times my heart beats fast, and I feel like I can't breathe, but I walk around outside, or just be still until it passes. My therapist says to stay present with it and the symptoms aren't as bad."

"Thanks, Gina. You did a wonderful job of documenting everything, and it helps me to understand how best to help you."

Gina's lack of sleep, that is, sleep deprivation, triggered the emotional processing part of her brain and set in motion brain wave patterns similar to people who worry too much, are anxious, or are prone to panic. As her sleep specialist, I saw clearly how vulnerable she was, and likely would become more so without sleep therapy. The insomnia prevents the appropriate emotional processing.

"Gina," I said, "I believe we can develop a helpful program for you. You have had a truly traumatic experience, and you have a temperament sensitive to stressors.

"You are so lucky that sleep medicine can offer you treatments, and coordinate it with your counselor when necessary to help you have the best first year of college you possibly can have!"

She looked up directly at my face and nodded again, this time with a wide smile and a bit of a sparkle in her eye.

I explained that her counselor would use some strategies from cognitive behavioral therapy such as imagery rehearsal therapy. I explained to Gina that the imagery she remembered of her event could continue to be distressing. To take charge of her toxic internal imagery and to reduce this distress, Gina and her therapist would rescript the images and create a new story. Imagery scripts follow a sequence like first finding a safe place, then relaxing, and then following the script the therapist voices for Gina to experience. The safe place is always an internal safe place, and then Gina can follow the script again at home. After rehearsing this rescripting of the nightmare, the disturbing dream begins to transform and lose its distressing properties.

Other techniques her therapist might use are journaling or a stress reduction program, which she knew about already. I further directed Gina to continue her sleep journal and check back with me about every three to four weeks as pharmacology also offered her some options.

What Is Post-Traumatic Stress Disorder (PTSD)?

PTSD is a medically recognized anxiety condition that occurs after witnessing or directly experiencing a life-threatening event. People have certainly been suffering from PTSD since humans walked the earth. However, the syndrome was not formally named until 1980, largely in response to the high numbers of Vietnam veterans who continued to suffer from battle fatigue long after they had returned home. "The estimated rate of lifetime PTSD among American Vietnam Veterans is about 30% for men and 27% for women."

Later, the definition expanded to include a delayed response to any traumatic event that continues to haunt the person and affect his or her life. PTSD is the only psychological disorder that does not originate within the patient, but from without. In fact, no one is diagnosed with PTSD unless he or she has experienced a highly traumatic event.

The types of recognized trauma are results of war, terrorism, violence and abuse, and natural disasters. An estimated two-thirds of the population is exposed to at least one such traumatic event in their lifetime. These experiences include the following:

1. **Developmental trauma** is a childhood experience of multiple or chronic exposures to interpersonal, adverse trauma, which could start at home with maltreatment or abuse. Children's trauma also includes medical procedures, community violence, and accidents.
2. **Acute trauma** is the result of the experiencer's subjective interpretation, the psychological state, in response to a terrifying event such as rape or other physical assault.
3. **Near-death experiences** include a dissociated state in which the experiencer feels disconnected from the body. Positive perceptions, such as the incident being spiritual, help, but do not mitigate the eventual appearance of PTSD symptoms, especially if the NDE occurs through a traumatic event such as an auto accident or surgery.
4. **Natural disasters** of late include Hurricane Katrina, the massive Sandy Hook storm, and the powerful tornadoes in Oklahoma.

5. **Long-term, chronic stress** is a condition of sustained, high levels of stress hormones, which eventually affect sleep, the cardiovascular and respiratory systems, as well as physically changing portions of the brain.

People from all walks of life can have PTSD and therefore PTSD-related sleep disorders, of which the highest prevalence is those who have experienced military combat. Recent studies show high rates of sleep disorders in military personnel, who may receive a co-existing diagnosis of a specific sleep disorder like insomnia or sleep apnea. An estimated one out of nine soldiers returning from Afghanistan and one out of six returning from Iraq have exhibited symptoms of PSTD.

A person with PTSD may relive the trauma through nightmares or intrusive thoughts. Persistent daytime recollections intrude into daytime consciousness. Such thoughts can be absent for a period and then savagely return at any time. Most persons with PTSD re-experience the trauma within the first year after the event.

PTSD sufferers tend to withdraw emotionally and avoid situations, places, and people, even thoughts perceived to be trauma triggers. Persons with PTSD show increased arousal, which can present as a range of symptoms from general irritability to hyperarousal as manifested by being sleepless. The fight-or-flight alert condition of the nervous system and metabolism contributes to nightmares and insomnia, and results in symptoms while both asleep and awake.

During waking hours, PTSD sufferers can continue to re-experience the trauma and remain hypersensitive to stimuli, particularly those that trigger memories of the event. Most likely, each of us has watched a television show where a combat veteran hears a car backfire and drops to the ground reliving a memory of combat gunfire or an explosion. Yet, a memory of trauma can include a car driver shaking and sweating with heart palpitations when approaching an intersection where she was involved in a severe car accident. Whatever the event, people feel a lingering sense of dread and fear, helplessness, and even horror long after the event has occurred.

The re-experience symptoms are also problematic during sleep. People may show complex motor behaviors and vocalizations as if reliving the event or acting out the incident. The sleeper can experience nightmares, nocturnal anxiety, panic attacks, hyperarousal, and sleeping difficulties.

The more common, self-reported sleep complaints by PTSD sufferers are

1. That 70% to 91% of patients with PTSD have difficulty falling or staying asleep
2. Inability to go to sleep
3. Frequent awakenings and then difficulty returning to sleep
4. Shorter sleep time
5. Nightmares
6. Anxiety dreams
7. Restless sleep
8. Daytime sleepiness

A research review correlated that insomnia and nightmares were the most prominent reported sleep issues of PTSD. The overall evidence of the hyperarousal mechanism in PTSD patients contributing to the listed sleep disruptions is strong. Recent studies have shown that patients with PTSD have elevated levels of a neurotransmitter called norepinephrine and that high levels following emotional trauma is a significant contributor to both daytime and nighttime problems. Norepinephrine, a stress hormone, is like adrenaline, in that it makes available to the body and brain the energy to be awake, alert, and ready for . . . whatever! This causes hyperarousal and disrupts rapid eye movement (REM) sleep.

In addition to the above symptoms, PTSD can also lead to a host of secondary problems, which contribute to sleep problems in going to sleep and maintaining sleep, including:

1. Panic attacks, social anxiety, conduct disorders, dissociation, and eating disorders
2. Low self-esteem, alcohol and substance abuse, problems at work, even arrest
3. Self-destructiveness, including risky sexual behavior, self-injury, and attempted suicide
4. Chronic physical ailments, including headaches, digestive problems, pain in the chest or other areas of the body

PTSD Checklist

To treat PTSD-related sleep disorders, a professional must first diagnose the disorder. If you believe that you or someone you know is suffering from PTSD, this checklist may help you decide to get a diagnosis immediately. Sleep disorders, insomnia, and excessive daytime sleepiness, even within a month after a traumatic event, are important predictors for the development of PTSD.

1. Have you suffered a traumatic experience that you keep reliving?
2. Do you feel a sense of numbness or emotional detachment?
3. Do you find yourself avoiding situations or activities that remind you of the trauma?
4. Are you suffering from insomnia or any other sleep disturbances, such as apnea?
5. Do you have frequent nightmares?

6. Do you have marital or other relationship difficulties?
7. Do you experience emotional instability?

Why It's Important to Resolve Sleep Disorders Related to PTSD

Because sleep complaints are high in deployed soldiers, one group of researchers set out to determine the prevalence of sleep disorders in combat-related PTSD and traumatic brain injury (TBI). The conclusion was that soldiers with combat-related PTSD and TBI did have high rates of sleep disorders and these were considered critical due to the chronic nature and high incidence rates.

1. In soldiers with blunt trauma, higher rates of obstructive sleep apnea were noted.
2. Soldiers with blast trauma had higher rates of insomnia.
3. Soldiers with PTSD, but without injuries, had higher rates of obstructive sleep apnea. This provided further possibility that sleep apnea was a preexisting disorder to PTSD in the combat soldiers.

Some people may have difficulty understanding the important significance of the rejuvenation and healing that occurs during sleep for patients with PTSD. Normal dreaming REM sleep is needed to cope with emotional trauma and is integrally involved in a process called fear extinction. In fear extinction, the brain uncouples the traumatic feelings associated with the original event from events common in everyday life.

We process the events of our day during sleep mainly through the limbic system. The amygdala are almond-shaped clusters of nuclei located in the medial temporal lobes of the brain and are responsible for memory consolidation, including forming long-term memories and processing emotional responses. The amygdala receives data about the day's events, and then sends it to the hippocampus for processing. The hippocampus checks these events against prior memories, and if it finds them similarly stressful, it tells the sympathetic nervous system to deal with the perceived threat. This initiates release of more stress hormones and more arousal, resulting in disrupted sleep.

It's imperative to resolve sleep disorders in those with PTSD for the purpose of healing the emotional trauma patterns that can occur during healthy sleep. Moreover, continued lack of sleep exacerbates stressors and leads to other health issues, as well making the sleep–wake cycle more problematic.

Treating Sleep Apnea Improves PTSD Symptoms

John was a 25-year-old combat veteran of Afghanistan sent to me for sleep apnea by the local VA hospital. He was withdrawn and unemotional. As we spoke I discovered he had severe insomnia and recurrent nightmares. He was becoming progressively more withdrawn, and he absolutely refused to go to certain places such as shopping malls. Large crowds and incessant noise brought back stressful emotions and even flashbacks of the war. John had PTSD.

The VA physician had prescribed some anti-anxiety medications, but John's sleep-related problems were not being addressed until he came to the Sleep Disorders Clinic. Because of John's loud snoring, I scheduled him for a sleep study. The sleep study revealed that John had sleep apnea. Interestingly, it also showed a pattern during REM sleep called fragmentation, during which there were numerous arousals, reducing the total amount of time spent in REM sleep. This is a pattern I frequently observe in PTSD patients. In fact, it may explain their inability to reconcile negative emotions because this fragmentation interrupts the duration of the REM sleep cycle.

John started on CPAP, and there was improvement in his daily functioning. He was less irritable and able to go out more often. However, his nightmares continued with little improvement. At that point, I elected to start him on a medication called prazosin. His response was excellent, and he stopped having nightmares after four weeks of treatment.

A high incidence of sleep apnea occurs in people with anxiety disorders, such as PTSD, generalized anxiety disorder and panic disorder, as well as obsessive–compulsive disorder. Sleep apnea has been noted most often in PTSD in returning veterans as well as in women who have suffered sexual trauma. This fact is not coincidental because the percent with sleep apnea in those groups with PTSD, especially the veterans, far exceeds what would be expected in a control group of similar sex and age. Sleep experts have learned that sleep apnea may be a preexisting condition, and, in many cases, treating the sleep disorder results in significant improvement in the anxiety disorders. Sleep apnea may actually intensify symptoms of PTSD.

Several recent studies have confirmed what sleep experts already thought to be true. Treating sleep apnea in PTSD with CPAP decreases and can even eliminate recurrent nightmares. Most likely, this can happen because untreated sleep apnea fragments REM sleep more than any other stage of sleep. This fragmenting inhibits the individual's ability to process and reconcile the trauma and results in continued nightmares.

Insomnia and Short Sleep Duration in PTSD

The first large-scale study (published 2010) of sleep patterns in 41,225 military personnel deployed to Iraq and

Afghanistan revealed that deployment definitely affected the veterans' sleep patterns. Results showed 25% reported sleep problems before deployment and a majority developed them during or after deployment.

Average reported sleep time was six and one-half hours, which the authors felt was restricted sleep time with a lasting impact on performance and mental health. A subgroup of post-deployed women, pregnant or new mothers, and moms of young children, was less than six hours. When compared to civilian pregnant mothers, the military moms slept less.

More recently, the results of later large-scale research provided a very different viewpoint about how lack of sleep affected mental health in military personnel. The findings of this study were part of a larger epidemiological investigation called the Millennium Cohort Study that included 15,204 servicemen and woman prior to first deployment. According to the study, military members who have insomnia symptoms before they deploy are more likely to develop mental health issues, which include depression, PTSD, panic, and anxiety. The odds to which insomnia predisposes service personnel to PTSD was described as equal to combat exposure. The conclusion was that insomnia itself is a risk factor for mental health problems, as well as being a symptom. This is more than a significant result, as it now sets the standard for further studies in determining if the chicken or the egg came first in terms of insomnia effects.

Moreover, researchers found that short sleep duration, defined as less than six hours per night, also increased the likelihood of developing PTSD. If you remember from the insomnia section, this sleep disorder is characterized by difficulty falling asleep and staying asleep. Short duration of sleep does not allow the sleeper to move through the necessary sleep cycles in order to restore balance, hormones, and other benefits of seven to nine hours of sleep. Think of the high school student Gina during the assault. Her physiological responses to the event included high levels of the brain neurotransmitter norepinephrine, causing hyperarousal and disrupting REM sleep.

Nightmares

Nightmares disturb sleep, which disrupts the REM sleep that stimulates the areas of the brain used in emotional processing. The consideration of nightmares and insomnia as hallmarks of PTSD is that sleep disruptions and shorter sleep durations develop into a cycle that exacerbates trauma and the ability to function well on a daily basis. Normal, uninterrupted REM sleep also enables the strengthening of fear extinction memory. Consistently disrupted REM sleep compromises fear extinction and recovery from PTSD.

Help for Sleep-Related PTSD Issues

Until recently, most therapies for PTSD were aimed at the daytime experience but ignored sleep problems. We now know that sleep problems must be addressed. When diagnosed with PTSD, there are a number of courses for treatment.

1. Treating sleep apnea, which appears to be present in higher-than-expected numbers with PTSD, can decrease sleep disruption and nightmares.
2. Treating insomnia and other sleep-disorder symptoms does help alleviate the waking symptoms of PTSD.

3. A technique called imagery rehearsal therapy has been very effective. The person with PTSD writes down the nightmare and then rewrites the script to be an unthreatening scenario that he or she rehearses during the day.
4. Cognitive behavioral therapy used to help those with insomnia without PTSD has proven to be beneficial.
5. Finally, several medications have been used to improve sleep and reduce nightmares. One in particular called *prazosin*, which blocks the effects of norepinephrine, has been effective.

The take home message for those with PTSD and for friends and family members is that the sleep issues associated with the disorder need to be addressed. The good news is that we are gaining better understanding into the mechanisms and effects of dysfunctional sleep in PTSD sufferers, and as a result, are developing new and effective treatments.

Answers to Your Questions

IS SLEEP APNEA COMMON?

Q. My son returned from Iraq a few years ago, and the VA diagnosed him with PTSD. He snores and the doctor was concerned he may have sleep apnea. They want him studied and treated if he has it. The VA doctor told him that sleep apnea seems to be very common in veterans with PTSD. Why would that be?

A. We are not sure, but in most studies, the incidence of sleep apnea is much higher than it is in men and women of a similar age and weight. One theory is that the sleep apnea was present before the PTSD. It is felt that by disrupting sleep repeatedly, sleep apnea makes it more difficult to deal with the emotional trauma associated with the PTSD. As a result, people with sleep apnea are more likely to go on to develop PTSD.

VIETNAM VETERAN STILL HAS NIGHTMARES

Q. My husband is a Vietnam war veteran. It has been over 40 years since he returned from the war, but he still has weekly nightmares. He goes for counseling, but it has not helped. Do you have any ideas?

A. Yes, several medications have been used to treat nightmare disorder in PTSD. The newer atypical antipsychotics such as Seroquel have been used with some success. However, ironically, an older blood pressure medication called prazosin has been the most successful. I would discuss this with your health care provider.

SLEEP STUDY OKAY?

Q. I am a 61-year-old Vietnam veteran. I have PTSD. I am a very light sleeper and always feel fatigued. The VA wants me to get a sleep study. What is the point, since most of us vets with PTSD sleep poorly?

A. Recent studies have shown that people with PTSD have a higher incidence of sleep-disordered breathing than normal. Most importantly, these studies demonstrated that spending much of the night in lighter stages of sleep—as is common in PTSD—can predispose one to sleep apnea. I would advise you to get the study done. At our sleep center, we have seen dramatic improvements in patients with PTSD after they are treated for their sleep-disordered breathing.

HOW LONG WILL VIETNAM NIGHTMARES CONTINUE?

Q. My husband is a Vietnam veteran. He was diagnosed with PTSD more than 20 years ago. He still has the same recurrent nightmare a few times a week. How long can this go on?

A. Actually, for a lifetime. A study done several years ago on World War II veterans showed recurrent nightmares in 60% of the subjects after 40 years. The good news is that there are some new pharmaceuticals and behavioral techniques available.

SERTRALINE

Q. I am an Iraq war veteran with PTSD. I am on a drug called sertraline and have done well. I no longer have flashbacks and feel calmer. However, my sleep problems such as insomnia and nightmares are still a problem. Shouldn't the sertraline have cured that as well?

A. Actually, that is not always the case. Many patients with PTSD have a high incidence of sleep disorders predating the PTSD. Sleep apnea, insomnia, and nightmare disorders seem to be higher in those with PTSD before it occurs. The theory is that poor sleep quality impairs emotional coping and may make these folks more susceptible to PTSD following severe emotional trauma. Recent studies have shown that sleep disorders may persist well after the PTSD has resolved. The trend in sleep medicine is to address the sleep issues as independent problems and not to automatically expect them to resolve when the PTSD improves. If this continues, consult with your health care provider. You may need a referral to someone familiar with these problems and its treatment, such as a sleep medicine specialist or psychiatrist.

WHAT WORKS?

Q. I am a Vietnam veteran. I was diagnosed with PTSD several years ago and attend a support group at the local VA hospital. It has helped, but I am still having trouble sleeping. It is difficult to fall and stay asleep. Worst of all, I have recurrent nightmares that have plagued me since the war. These group sessions do not seem to be helping me with my sleep. Do you have any suggestions for me?

A. Yes, I do. We know that people with PTSD have sleep-related problems. Recurrent nightmares are a major issue. Recent studies have shown that patients with PTSD have elevated levels of a neurotransmitter called norepinephrine. We have found that a blood pressure medication called prazosin that blocks norepinephrine in the brain has been effective in eliminating sleep problems in PTSD. You should discuss this with your health care provider.

GOOD SLEEP, BAD MOODS

Q. My brother lives with us. He came back from Iraq with PTSD. He is having trouble falling and staying asleep, which is making him increasingly irritable. I am trying to get him to seek help. Do you think it would make a difference?

A. The answer is yes. Insomnia is an integral problem associated with PTSD. If untreated, it interferes with emotional adaptation and further contributes to the increased irritability associated with PTSD. The good news is that there are now treatment options, both behavioral and pharmacological. To help with the sleep disorders associated with PTSD, I would urge your brother to seek help from the Veterans Administration or your family physician.

PTSD FROM CAR ACCIDENT

Q. My husband was in a terrible car accident several years ago. He was diagnosed with PTSD about a year later. Unfortunately, he still wakes up in a panic with nightmares about the accident. Is there anything that can be done about this? He has undergone therapy and most of the other symptoms have resolved.

A: Yes, there is hope for those with recurrent nightmares in PTSD. The nightmares are the re-experiencing of the event during sleep. There are both pharmaceutical and behavioral treatments available. Among the medications, an older blood pressure medication called prazosin seems to be the best. Imagery rehearsal therapy is a cognitive treatment. In this therapy, the person alters the disturbing content of the dream to a more pleasant one and rehearses the change in their mind during the day. It has been shown to be very effective in studies done with military veterans.

13

Sleep Disorders and ADHD

Sleep is the golden chain that ties health and our bodies together.

—THOMAS DEKKER

The estimated percentage of children and adolescents in the United States diagnosed with attention deficit hyperactivity disorder (ADHD) is 5.9% to 7.1%, and the numbers continue to rise. Symptoms, including difficulty staying focused and paying attention, difficulty controlling behavior, and hyperactivity (overactivity), often continue into adulthood. A long-term study following young children (three to four years old) diagnosed early with ADHD and treated through educational and pharmaceutical methods found that from 30% to 70% still experienced symptoms as adults. Their symptoms persisted because there is a significant, deeper issue at play. Many kids and adults with ADHD have an underlying sleep disorder. Sleep problems can exacerbate ADHD symptoms and treating the sleep disorder will improve the ADHD symptoms. Conversely, some children are misdiagnosed with ADHD when the cause of their symptoms is an untreated sleep disorder, like sleep apnea, restless legs syndrome (RLS), or inadequate sleep.

Children, Sleep, and ADHD

In my sleep practice, I see many caring parents who are unaware of how much sleep children require. It is estimated that 30% of children demonstrate symptoms of sleep disorders. Children need 11 to 12 hours of sleep every night. Deprived these hours, they become irritable, have difficulty sitting still, and have a hard time concentrating. One sleep study involving 2,463 children of 6 to 15 years old, showed

- Sleep problems are more likely to cause children to be inattentive, hyperactive, impulsive, and display opposi-tional behaviors.
- As a result of being sleepy, children may be moody, emo-tionally explosive, and/or aggressive.

Lack of sleep also affects their cognitive development. In a study reported in the British *Journal of Epidemiology and Community Health,* children who demonstrated irregular bedtimes up to the age of three were the most negatively affected when it came to reading, math skills, and spatial awareness. When followed over time, the same children con-tinued to lag developmentally, even at the age of seven—and girls more than boys. The authors concluded that the first three years of life seem to be a particularly sensitive time for sleep and its relationship to cognitive development.

A more recent study published in the *Journal of Pediatric Psychology* further verified the impact of lack of sleep on children's emotions and cognitive performance. In the study, 32 children (8 to 12 years old) wore devices that could detect sleep, called actigraphs. These were worn on the wrist, similarly to a watch. They detected motion or its absence and could differentiate between being asleep and being awake. The children were initially studied under their usual sleep habits for one week. Then during week two, half were deprived of one hour of sleep and the other half had their sleep lengthened by one hour. During week three, each group was exposed to the opposite condition.

The study period ended on a Friday. The following morning the children were put through a number of tests of cognitive function such as short-term and working memory. They were also tested for emotional responses to positive and negative images. The parents filled out detailed questionnaires about their children's cognitive ability and emotional responses during the test period.

The results were quite impressive. Parents reported that their children had more difficulty regulating their emotions when they were in the short-sleep compared to the long-sleep duration group. In addition, the children, when tested, expressed far fewer positive responses to various stimuli when they were in the short-sleep group.

Additionally, short-term and working memory, as well as math fluency, were found to be negatively affected in the short-sleep group. Both parental observations and testing demonstrated significant problems with attention as well.

As you can see from the previously mentioned studies, many of these symptoms that children exhibited due to lack of sleep were similar to symptoms for ADHD, and could complicate an accurate ADHD diagnosis. The following table compares symptoms of children with ADHD to children with sleep disorders.

Children with ADHD Diagnosis	Children with Sleep Disorders
Difficulty paying attention; trouble maintaining consistent focus	Easily distracted, not thinking clearly
Difficulty remembering, forgetful	Problems concentrating, learning, and remembering
Disorganized	
Need to move or fidget, run or be on the go without direction or attention to environment	Prone to accidents
Slower motor response	Slower reaction time
Impulsive or hyperactive	Moody or emotional
	Behavioral issues of resistance exacerbated by sleep disruptions, inattention, or emotional over-reactivity

Some researchers believe that the presence of sleep problems can be a predictor for ADHD. A recently published comprehensive study investigated sleep duration and disturbance as predictors of ADHD diagnoses in children from birth through age 11. Of the assessed 8,195 children, 173 children (2.1%) met the criteria for ADHD. According to the study, ADHD children had more night awakenings than their peers at every age. Shorter sleep durations and disruptions appeared early and are a significant predictor of ADHD between ages three and five.

A child diagnosed with ADHD is likely to have a sleep disorder. The most common issues include excessive daytime sleepiness, trouble falling asleep, difficulties awakening, restless legs syndrome, and sleep apnea. In a vicious cycle, the sleep problem aggravates the ADHD symptoms and ADHD behaviors in children can reinforce sleep issues. The good news is that when the children's sleep disorders received treatment, the ADHD symptoms improved. For example, attention deficits were reported in up to 95% of obstructive sleep apnea (OSA) patients. In patients with the full ADHD syndrome, 20% to 30% showed incidence of OSA. After treatment for the sleep apnea, behavior and attention improved.

The Most Common Sleep Disorders Associated with ADHD

The most common sleep disorders that coexist with ADHD in children are:

1. Higher daytime sleepiness.
2. More movements in sleep.
3. Sleep-disordered breathing, sleep apnea, and sleep hypopnea, which is a partial obstruction to breathing resulting in at least a 3% drop in oxygen saturation. It is considered just as deleterious as an apnea.

DAYTIME SLEEPINESS

ADHD children have difficulty staying awake during the day. Dr. Thomas Brown indicates that daytime drowsiness afflicts many with ADHD. Brown writes, "Many with ADD [ADHD] syndrome report that they are often tired during the day because they have chronic and severe difficulties in settling into sleep, even when they are very tired and want to fall asleep."

If a child is excessively sleepy, the diagnosis may be narcolepsy. Unfortunately, the diagnosis of narcolepsy is frequently delayed by 10 or more years because the symptoms are frequently misattributed to some other disorder.

MORE MOVEMENT IN SLEEP: RESTLESS LEGS SYNDROME

Restless legs syndrome (RLS) refers to uncomfortable, even painful sensations in the legs that can itch, tingle, or feel like ants crawling on you. Mostly occurring in the evening, the solution is movement. RLS can occur with periodic leg movement. This syndrome can often be alleviated with iron supplements as it is related to low iron. Remember that 20% of adults recall having symptoms of restless legs as kids.

Children with RLS can present with symptoms that are hard to differentiate from ADHD. Many have a hard time relating what they are feeling, or are misdiagnosed as having "growing pains." Their leg pain can deprive them of much needed sleep at night or make it impossible to sit still in class during the day.

These children not only move upper and lower limbs more frequently during the night, but also for longer periods. A cross-sectional survey of 866 children with ADHD symptoms, as well as RLS symptoms, showed the two symptoms were twice as likely to occur together than just by chance. Also, parents have reported during the years that their ADHD children displayed restless legs syndrome and periodic limb movement (PLM) during the day as well as at night.

Children with ADHD have an increased prevalence of PLMs and children with PLM disorders are more likely to have ADHD. PLMs are movements of the legs (and occasionally the upper limbs) that occur after falling asleep. Although very common in children with restless legs syndrome, they are not considered to be the same thing. RLS is a conscious discomfort. PLM occurs while sleeping and the individual is not aware. Treatment of PLM with dopamine agonists, a compound that activates dopamine receptors when dopamine is absent, improved sleep quality, sleep quantity, and also ADHD symptoms.

SLEEP-DISORDERED BREATHING, SLEEP APNEA, AND HYPOPNEA

This group of disorders includes abnormalities of breathing patterns like pauses in breathing while sleeping. In children, the two primary sleep breathing issues are snoring and OSA. Three to twelve percent of children have incidents of habitual snoring. Of those who snore, 1% to 3% are most likely have sleep apnea. OSA, the most common type of sleep apnea, is caused by obstruction of the upper airway and is characterized by repetitive pauses in breathing during sleep, typically last 10 to 40 seconds, and a reduction in blood oxygen saturation. Children with OSA often behave as if overtired: moody, aggressive, or hyperactive.

The good news is that OSA-diagnosed children's academic functioning improved with an adenotonsillectomy compared with children who were not treated. A recent NIH-sponsored study called the Childhood Adenotonsillectomy Trial (CHAT) addressed this issue. For seven months, researchers followed 464 children who were five to nine years old. All of the children had mild to moderate sleep apnea, and they were placed in one of two groups, for surgery or for "watchful waiting." Those children who underwent the surgical procedure did better regarding impulsivity, restlessness, and emotional lability. They also slept better and were less sleepy and fatigued than the control group. Surprisingly, this study failed to demonstrate improvements in cognition although several studies have made this point.

This procedure helped my patient Sam, a pale-faced, thin nine-year-old child with a head of blonde curls. At our first meeting, he walked up to me, shook my hand, and in a West Texas drawl said, "Hiya, doctor. I'm Samuel James Buford thuh third. I'm here fer yer help!"

I noticed his mom. "Hello, Mrs. Buford, please have a seat. And Samuel James Buford, what name shall I call you?"

"Ya really wanna know?"

"Yes, of course."

"Ya know all of us from West Texas have two names. Mom's is Carla Lou, and mine is Sammy Jim." Saying "Sammy Jim" with the straightest face I bet he practiced all morning cracked the façade. The giddy boy was animated in laughing, high-fiving his knee several times, and bouncing into his chair next to his mother. The legs started swinging as if he were kicking air.

Sammy's medical file indicated he was recently referred to the school psychologist for an evaluation of possible ADHD. Records described him as hyperactive with a penchant for practical jokes, which apparently still gets him into trouble. He appears to be bright according to his school's test scores. His medical history also indicated he had the normal "going to school" childhood bouts with chicken pox, strep throat, and a cold or two. The family doctor wondered about a sleep issue for the snoring and hyperactivity.

"Mrs. Buford, how can I help you and Sammy Jim today? "

"Sammy Jim's teacher believes he needs to be checked for a sleep disorder after she read a news article. The possible confusion of symptoms between sleep and ADHD interested her. I wrote down what she referred to right here: 'The symptoms of sleep deprivation in children resemble those of ADHD. While adults experience sleep deprivation as drowsiness and sluggishness, sleepless children often become wired, moody, and obstinate. They may have trouble focusing, sitting still and getting along with peers.' All of those symptoms except moody and obstinate describe Sammy Jim."

I asked Mrs. Buford to complete my checklist of symptoms for children. Her responses are below:

DR. ROSENBERG'S CHECKLIST FOR PRESCHOOL AND SCHOOL-AGED CHILDREN

Question	Parent's Answer
What time does child go to bed?	Between 9:00 and 10:00 p.m.
What is routine after dinner and before bed?	Helps with dishes. Completes homework. Might watch a TV show before bed. Maybe showers or brushes teeth and goes to bed.
Is child reluctant to go to bed?	Not usually—and sometimes wants a Game Boy.
Does child ask continuously for something before lights out?	No.

(continued)

DR. ROSENBERG'S CHECKLIST FOR PRESCHOOL AND SCHOOL-AGED CHILDREN

(continued)

Question	Parent's Answer
Does child wake frequently, and how often, during night?	Yes, Sam wakes up around several times at night. Maybe four times a week.
How long does it take your child to go back to sleep?	Maybe about 30 minutes.
Does child get up early?	Not usually.
Does child cry out during the night?	No.
How does parent respond each night to awakenings or crying out?	Gets up to check on son when hears him stirring.
What kind of bed does your child sleep in?	Regular single bed.
Is the room prepared for sleep? (dark, cool, quiet, without distractions)	Yes, except for Nintendo Game Boy.
Does your child sleep with a favorite. . . .?	Just the Game Boy.
Does your child ever sleep with you? How often? Under what circumstances?	No.
Is your child restless during sleep? How?	Not in any unusual way.
Does your child snore?	Yes, every night. Mostly the snoring is soft and only occasionally loud.
Does your child appear to struggle to breathe while sleeping?	Don't see struggling.
Is your child a restless sleeper, constantly moving his legs while asleep?	Yes.
Does your child complain of pain such as cramps or owies in his legs at night?	No.

(continued)

DR. ROSENBERG'S CHECKLIST FOR PRESCHOOL AND SCHOOL-AGED CHILDREN
(continued)

Question	Parent's Answer
Do you find your child wandering the house after everyone has gone to bed?	No.
Is your child sleepier during the day than peers his or her age?	Seems so, hard to judge.

Because of Sammy Jim's habitual snoring, I became suspicious that he might have sleep apnea. After all, the American Academy of Pediatrics recommends children be tested for sleep apnea if they snore chronically. We proceeded with a sleep study in the lab that confirmed Sam had sleep apnea. In fact, he stopped breathing about 16 times an hour. This would be considered moderate in an adult but indicates severity in a child. We also found that as a result of these episodes Sam's blood oxygen saturations dropped periodically with each event.

I had noticed during the physical exam that Sam had enlarged tonsils. I rated them a 3 to 4 on a scale of 4 that we use. As a result, I suggested Mrs. Buford consult with an ear, nose, and throat doctor as Sam seemed to be a good candidate for an adenotonsillectomy. Sam underwent the surgery and about eight weeks later, when he had healed, we retested him. He showed enough improvement that we did not need to proceed with continuous positive airway pressure therapy (CPAP) as a treatment.

ADOLESCENTS AND ADULTS

For people diagnosed with ADHD in adulthood, misdiagnosis due to an unrecognized sleep disorder is a possibility. In one study, researchers compared narcolepsy (a neurological sleep disorder with disturbed nocturnal sleep and an abnormal daytime sleep pattern), idiopathic hypersomnia (thought to be a neurological disorder, characterized primarily by severe excessive daytime sleepiness), and ADHD, and found a high percentage of overlapping symptoms, suggesting the possibility of adult ADHD misdiagnosis.

Adolescents and adults with ADHD are very restless sleepers with active movements like turning. They have a higher incidence of sleep-onset insomnia (going to sleep) and sleep-maintenance insomnia (staying asleep). The most common sleep problems reported are:

- Insomnia. Adults with ADHD have a higher than normal incidence of insomnia.
- Being restless—kicking, tossing, and turning. One study concluded that symptoms of ADHD are more common in RLS patients than in patients with insomnia. RLS and ADHD may be part of a single symptom complex, and dopamine deficiency may play a role in both disorders.
- Difficulty waking up as a chronic problem, even if they felt they had a good night's sleep.
- Sleep apnea.

Some adults with ADHD symptoms become alert as the day progresses and are more ready to work or socialize in the evening, delaying their sleep onset as well as their ability to awaken the next morning. These sleep–wake problems can be attributed to significant changes in the circadian rhythms of adults with ADHD. As compared with control groups, adults with ADHD show decreased sleep duration and reduced quality of sleep.

Cortisol levels are also a factor. Cortisol is usually high when we are awake, alert, or working. For most people, cortisol levels are at their lowest at 11:00 p.m. and highest at 9:00 a.m. For those with ADHD, cortisol levels peak toward evening when they should be dropping. This also delays the production of melatonin, a hormone that promotes sleep. Melatonin supplements proved effective in helping my patient James.

James was 42 years old and appeared to be moderately obese. James had a fairly successful business, but had a hard time focusing and tended to lose interest in things quickly. James explained that he had been diagnosed with adult ADHD seven years prior and was taking Adderall. He described himself at work as hyperfocused to the exclusion of everything and everyone else.

I noticed when James and his wife sat down in my office that his legs were moving after a short time. I guessed he had a hard time staying still and was more restless than relaxed at home also. During our initial conversation about his sleeping patterns, I watched him impulsively jump into my sentences with "Let me explain . . ." or "I think. . . ."

James described his sleep problems as trouble falling asleep and further difficulty staying asleep. I attributed some of this to his moderate obesity. Then I questioned his wife and she said, "He snores." That's when we started talking about scheduling James for a sleep study. I advised him to get a diagnostic polysomnogram in the sleep lab, and the results showed that he did have sleep apnea.

He went on CPAP and has shown significant improvement. He no longer wakes in the middle of the night, suggesting his inability to remain asleep had to do with the sleep apnea. His ability to stay asleep has improved by taking melatonin about one to two hours before going to bed. Now, he is less sleepy and better functioning during his workday.

TREATMENT OPTIONS

There is a good chance that by addressing your sleep problems, you will improve your ADHD.

Trouble getting to sleep: Practice good sleep hygiene, especially eliminating all sources of blue light (computers, televisions, and other electronic devices). Consider taking a low trial dose of melatonin, 1 to 3 milligrams, an hour or two before bed. Insomnia could also be related to medications you may be taking for ADHD. Ritalin, Adderall, and dextroamphetamine are commonly used in ADHD and all cause insomnia, especially if dosing is too close to bedtime. Discuss options with your health care provider.

Trouble staying asleep: A sign of an underlying sleep disorder, such as insomnia.

Early morning awakenings: Rule out depression as part of the problem.

Snoring: A sign of possible sleep apnea. Speak with a sleep specialist. Sleep apnea treatment can yield significant improvement.

Discomfort in the extremities, usually the legs: If movement relieves discomfort, then it may be RLS. Antidepressants, antipsychotics, and over-the-counter sleep aids that contain diphenhydramine can cause or exacerbate RLS. Low iron levels are also a cause; have your doctor check your iron levels with a test called ferritin. If none of these predisposing conditions are found, then treatment with medications for RLS is very effective.

Answers to Your Questions

SLEEP APNEA AND ADHD

Q. My six-year-old has sleep apnea. I have been told that he should have his tonsils and adenoids removed, but I am a bit reluctant to do this. What type of benefit might he get from having this done? He is somewhat hyperactive.

A. A recent study, funded by the NIH, involved 464 children. The study demonstrated the benefits of surgery in children with sleep apnea. Children who underwent surgery showed improvement in sleep quality, impulse control, and quality of life. Beneficial effects were observed, even among overweight children in whom there has been particular uncertainty about the role of surgery. I hope that answers your question.

SLEEPINESS

Q. My nine-year-old granddaughter was diagnosed with ADHD. She only sleeps seven hours a night. I know that can't be enough. Can it be contributing to the ADHD?

A. Yes, it may be a contributing factor. Recent studies have shown that we need a proper amount of sleep for our memory to function during the day. In fact, the type of memory called declarative is particularly abnormal in ADHD. Declarative memory is particularly dependent on slow wave sleep (deep sleep). If this is impaired because of lack of sleep, it may further inhibit the ability to learn. So it is very important that children with ADHD get enough sleep. A nine-year-old requires at least 10 hours of sleep each night.

Self-Check: Your Child's Sleep Habits

Our job as parents and professionals is to be aware of children's sleep needs and sleep habits. If left untreated, sleep problems suffered in childhood will persist into adolescence and adulthood. It's imperative to treat childhood sleep problems early, especially if the child has ADHD. In many instances, dealing with a child's sleep problem will improve his or her ADHD. If you have a child with ADHD, take the time to notice any of these behaviors:

- Snoring
- An inability to fall or stay asleep
- Complaints of always feeling tired and fatigued
- Frequent leg movements at rest or while asleep

If you suspect your child has a sleep disorder, schedule an appointment with a sleep doctor and use the checklist earlier in this chapter to help you discuss your child's symptoms.

Conclusion: Sleep Well

Start where you are.
Use what you have.
Do what you can.
—ARTHUR ASHE

Sleep . . . the time for you to balance the internal systems and recalibrate your circadian clock. You've now read how sleep is the healing elixir for emotional memories, a clear mind, and a positive mood. How ingenious of nature to provide sleep cycles to restore balance. Take the opportunity now to change what is not working for you. Make a positive intention to sleep well every night and feel great every day.

Start Where You Are

If changing your sleep hygiene and habits seems over-whelming, then start where you are. Choose your first step, close your eyes, and see yourself take that step successfully. Jenna had difficulty knowing what her first step would be after her husband died quite suddenly of an undiagnosed heart condition. They lived their dreams for seven years, and suddenly her greatest difficulty in sleeping in their bedroom was memories of her husband. She knew she had to firmly decide to take the first step of changing the room to suit her personality, changing out somber earth tone bedding and furniture that so suited her husband. She wanted bright blue skies, white walls, and soft bedding that hugged her to sleep. She wanted comfort, respite, and calm—the qualities her husband brought to their relationship. She took the first step of choosing her sleeping style.

Where will you start? Most people like to organize and prioritize. What can you organize now to make your sleeping space inviting? Is there clutter you want to clear? How about that lamp you don't like or the stack of books you haven't read yet? Clean this one sleeping space, and you'll be amazed at how inviting it feels to go to sleep now. Trust that the next step will be easier, and keep visualizing your deep, comfortable sleep.

Use What You Have

Are your nightly rituals a priority now that you understand how restorative sleep can improve how you feel? Use the new knowledge and checklists from this book to review your nightly rituals, eating habits, and any delay tactics that exacerbate your moods or actions. Put an end to the delayed sleep, the late night snacks, and the electronic games that keep you awake. Do you need to keep a sleep diary? Evaluate your diet before bed? Why not jot down some notes on using what you have to make your sleep better, and in another column, list what you would like or feel you need to sleep better: a different pillow, perhaps? A journal for listing negative thoughts? Or possibly a gratitude journal to review your day with a sense of fulfillment? What you have are qualities of common sense, knowing what you need to change, and the willingness to make that change. You have strength, and from this book you have knowledge to get a good night's sleep every night.

Do What You Can

In the Introduction, I mentioned that in the United States alone, 50 to 70 million people suffer from chronic sleep issues. The huge number astounds me because it presents a world health problem for this century. The adverse effects of sleep deprivation drain people's focus, energy, health, and optimism. The enormous importance of that sentence is brought home every time I see a patient succeed in his or her sleep programs. They never fail to share their success stories with others who also suffer from sleep disorders.

Will you do what you can to champion your sleep health as an example to others? When someone compliments you on your vitality and positivity, tell them how well you sleep and how you changed what wasn't working for your rest. Remember that 70 million people need an example of your boldness to stop what isn't working and start learning how a night of deep, fulfilling sleep can improve health. While this is the conclusion of this sleep book, it is the first step in your journey to better sleep, calmer emotions, and excellent health. Sleep well!

Appendices

Tools to support better sleep hygiene and to evaluate how you sleep:

Better Sleep Quick Reference

Attention Deficit Hyperactivity Disorder Checklist

Better Sleep Quick Reference

Good sleep practices are necessary to have normal, quality sleep time, and full alertness during the day. I recommend these better sleep guidelines:

1. **Get up and go to bed at the same time each day.**

   This practice may be difficult at first, especially given our busy and often erratic schedules. Yet those scheduled activities for work, school, exercise, errands, and family also help to regulate your internal body clock's time to go to bed at the same time each night. Adhering to a sleep routine helps to regulate our circadian rhythm. Be sure to stick with the schedule on the weekend, too. Staying up until 3:00 a.m. on Saturday night and sleeping in on Sunday may throw off the rhythm you established throughout the week.

2. **Make your bedroom conducive to sleep.**

   Studies show that it is easiest to fall asleep in a cool, quiet, and dark environment. I recommend your bedroom temperature remain around 68°F. Be sure to eliminate as much noise and light as possible. If it gets too warm, make sure you adjust the temperature and use a fan or air conditioner so that the heat does not wake you up in the middle of the night.

3. **Keep the electronics out of the bedroom and don't use them right before sleep.**

   It is very important to avoid television, electronic games, and computers right before going to bed. In fact, they should be kept out of the bedroom altogether. These things stimulate the brain and make it much more difficult to fall asleep. Even the light of a computer screen can keep your brain from relaxing. The same is true of

218 • • • APPENDICES

your cell phone. Even if the ringer is off, the light from the phone or the sound of it vibrating can interrupt your sleep. The light hitting the retina suppresses the production of your sleep hormone melatonin.

4. Avoid caffeine, alcohol, and nicotine four to six hours before bedtime.

It's not good enough to avoid that late night espresso. Any caffeine ingested in the late afternoon or early evening can affect your sleep. Remember that this stimulant is not only found in drinks such as coffee, soda, and tea, but it is also found in certain foods, such as chocolate.

Some people are surprised to learn that nicotine and even alcohol can disrupt sleep. While alcohol might make you feel drowsy initially, it just as easily interrupts the stages of sleep, even to the point where you get up in the middle of the night. As alcohol is metabolized and leaves your body, it causes a slight withdrawal characterized by an increase in activity of the sympathetic fight-or-flight nervous system and an elevation of the stress hormone cortisol.

5. Take a power nap for 30 minutes.

If you are sleep-deprived at night, you might want nothing more than to lie down during the day. Taking naps disrupts the natural drive to sleep at night, so in reality, you will only be perpetuating the cycle of insomnia. If you must nap, then take a power nap of no more than 30 minutes and not after 4:00 p.m. Otherwise, naps will decrease your brain's drive for sleep that night.

6. Remove the television from the bedroom.

Your bedroom should be a place for calmness and rest where you sleep or connect with your partner, only.

7. **Exercise each day, but avoid doing it four hours before bedtime.**

   Daily workouts have been shown to improve the quality of our sleep. But when you exercise within a few hours of bedtime, it will give you an energy boost that may prevent you from falling asleep. Exercising before sleep raises the core body temperature and elevates levels of cortisol and adrenaline, all of which prevent you from falling asleep.

8. **Create a healthy bedtime ritual.**

   Nightly relaxing rituals can help prepare the body and mind to get ready for sleep. Take at least 15 minutes at the end of each day to read a book, listen to relaxing music, or soak awhile in a warm bath.

9. **When you have trouble falling asleep, don't stress out.**

   Everyone has tossed and turned a few nights in their life. But if you are sleep-challenged, one of the worse things you can do is to force the issue. Eventually, you will associate bedtime with anxiety and that can actually make the problem worse. The best thing to do is to get up, go to another quiet area of the house, and try to relax. When you feel ready to fall asleep, then head back to the bedroom.

10. **Stop eating and drinking a few hours before going to bed.**

    You can be in the deepest sleep of your life, and still wake up from a full bladder. Also, if you have digestive problems such as heartburn or acid reflux, you are more likely to have an attack if you lie down so soon after eating.

11. **Ignore your to-do list.**

    Have you gone to bed and then suddenly remembered that important thing you forgot to take care of?

If you're one of those people who get out of bed to tackle the task, it's time to stop! Sleep must be your priority now. Realize that only so many things can get done in one day. Of course, if the task is important enough that *not* doing it will keep you awake, then take care of it as quickly as possible. Also, though recreation is important, be sure to limit any activities that would infringe on the new sleep schedule. Your first priority right now should be to get your sleep regulated, if only because being well-rested will enable you to enjoy your waking hours all the more.

Attention Deficit Hyperactivity Disorder Checklist

If you believe that a child in your family may have attention deficit hyperactivity disorder (ADHD), this very simplified checklist provides the behaviors most observed in children who eventually receive this diagnosis. ADHD is one of the more common neurobehavioral disorders in which children have trouble paying attention, controlling impulsivity (i.e., they may act without thinking about what the result will be), and in some cases, are overly active. Please note that at least half of the symptoms should be observed in one child before sharing the results with your doctor. A child with ADHD might have the following symptoms:

1. Has a hard time paying attention.
2. Daydreams a lot.
3. Does not seem to listen.
4. Is easily distracted from schoolwork or play.
5. Forgets things.
6. Is in constant motion or unable to stay seated.
7. Squirms or fidgets.
8. Talks too much.
9. May not be able to play quietly.
10. Acts and speaks without thinking.
11. Has trouble taking turns.
12. Interrupts others.

Glossary

Actigraphy—monitoring a patient's rest and movement periods through a small actigraph, which measures gross motor activity, worn on the patient's dominant arm.

Advanced Sleep Phase Syndrome (ASPS)—occurs when a person's "body clock" (i.e., circadian rhythm) is set to fall asleep very early in the evening. People who have ASPS tend to wake up very early, or in the middle of the night, and can't go back to sleep.

Antidepressants—drugs used to treat moderate or severe depression.

Apnea—complete cessation of airflow at the nose and/or mouth and lasting about 10 seconds.

Arousal—a physiological and psychological state of being awake or reactive to stimuli.

Attention-Deficit Hyperactivity Disorder (ADHD)—a common childhood, neurological disorder that can continue through adolescence and adulthood. Symptoms can include difficulty in staying focused, paying attention, controlling impulsivity, and hyperactivity.

Biological Clock—the groups of cells that regulate biological rhythms of sleeping/waking, reproductive cycles, and other aspects of biological timing.

Central Sleep Apnea (CSA)—a sleep-related disorder in which the effort to breathe is diminished or absent, typically for more than 30 seconds, either intermittently or in cycles called Cheyne–Stokes respiration, and is usually associated with a reduction in blood oxygen saturation.

Cerebral Cortex—the brain's outer layer of gray tissue that is responsible for higher nervous and cognitive functions.

Chronic Insomnia—a sleep disorder in which there is an inability to fall asleep or to stay asleep, or has early morning awakenings lasting at least three months and occurring a minimum of three days per week.

Chronobiology—the biological study of natural cycles (solar, lunar) and how one's circadian rhythms adapt.

Circadian Rhythm—24-hour periods or cycles of biological activity or function.

Circadian Rhythm Sleep Disorders—circadian rhythm disorders are disruptions in a person's circadian rhythm—a name given to the "internal body clock" that regulates the (approximately) 24-hour cycle of biological processes. The circadian sleep disorders refer to a continuous or occasional disruption of sleep patterns.

Cognitive Behavioral Therapy (CBT)—a psychotherapy approach that addresses dysfunctional emotions, maladaptive behaviors, and cognitive processes and contents. CBT refers to the combination of cognitive therapy and behavior therapy.

Cognitive Therapy—therapeutic approach used for transforming faulty beliefs and attitudes about sleep, insomnia, and the next-day consequences. The goal is to control intrusive thoughts at bedtime and prevent excessive monitoring of the daytime results of insomnia.

Complex Sleep Apnea (CSA)—a form of sleep apnea in which central apneas persist or emerge during attempts to treat obstructive sleep apnea with a continuous positive airway pressure (CPAP) or bi-level BiPAP device.

Confusional Arousal—a disorder associated with non-REM sleep in which a person appears mentally confused or demonstrates disoriented behavior during or following arousal, usually from slow-wave sleep.

CPAP—continuous positive airway pressure, a method of respiratory ventilation used primarily in the treatment of sleep apnea.

(Excessive) Daytime Sleepiness—being persistently sleepy, lacking energy, even after adequate sleep.

Delayed Sleep Phase Syndrome—circadian rhythm sleep disorder in which the sleep pattern is delayed two or more hours from a normal bedtime.

Delta Waves—brain waves with a frequency of 0 hertz to 4 hertz that emanate from the forward frontal lobes portion of the brain during deep sleep in normal adults.

Desynchronization—when the internal biological clocks are out of phase (or out of sync) with external or environmental signals.

Diurnal—active or occurring during the daytime; repeating once each 24 hours.

Dreaming—thoughts, feelings, or images that occur during sleep.

Dyssomnias—a category of sleep disorders that make it difficult to go to sleep or to stay asleep.

Electroencephalography (EEG)—a test that measures the brain's electrical activity.

Endocrine System—the body's system of glands that secrete hormones into the bloodstream.

Endogenous Rhythms—the internal rhythms driven by the self-sustaining biological clocks.

Entrain—to reset or align with the biological clock.

Enuresis—bed-wetting.

Exacerbate—to aggravate or make severity worse.

Executive Functions (Thinking Skills)—the mentation enabling a person to link past experiences with present actions such as planning, organizing, strategizing, paying attention to and remembering details, and managing time and space.

Exogenous Rhythms—rhythms that external cues directly regulate or influence. Cues are not generated internally.

Free-Running Disorder—a circadian sleep disorder in which environmental cues such as sunset for sleeping do not entrain sleep patterns.

Gene—a DNA sequence that encodes a protein.

Homeostasis—the ability of an organism or cell to maintain internal equilibrium by adjusting its internal processes.

Homeostatic Regulation of Sleep—the neurobiological signals mediating the pressure or urge to sleep.

Hypersomnia—sleep of excessive depth or abnormal duration, usually caused by psychological rather than physical factors and characterized by a state of confusion on awakening.

Hypersomnolence—excessive drowsiness.

Hypopnea—hypopnea is a 30% drop in flow lasting at least 10 seconds accompanied by a 3% drop in oxygen saturation or an arousal from sleep.

Hypothalamus—the part of the brain that lies below the thalamus and regulates body temperature and metabolic processes.

Insomnia—sleeplessness with chronic difficulty with sleep onset or maintenance of sleep, or a perception of non refreshing sleep.

Irregular Sleep–Wake Syndrome—a rare disorder of sleeping without a set schedule because of a problem with brain function or a problem with the body's circadian rhythms (internal clock).

Jet Lag Disorder—a change or disruption of normal circadian rhythms in transatlantic travel that results from a disparity between the internal clock and the external clock at your destination in desynchronizing the internal clock, as one passes through several time zones.

Kleine-Levin Syndrome—recurrent episodes of dramatic hypersomnia lasting from two days to several weeks. These episodes are associated with behavioral and cognitive abnormalities, binge eating, hypersexuality, and alternate with long asymptomatic periods that last months to years.

Melatonin—the pineal gland's secretion of a hormone derived from the amino acid tryptophan, and it synchronizes biological clock neurons in the suprachiasmatic nucleus.

Multiple Sleep Latency Test (MSLT)—a test for daytime sleepiness.

Narcolepsy—chronic sleep disorder characterized by excessive and overwhelming daytime sleepiness (even after adequate nighttime sleep) usually associated with a transient loss of muscle tone in response to emotions called cataplexy.

Neurotransmitter—a chemical produced by neurons that carries messages to other neurons.

Night (Nocturnal) Eating—the biological clock for eating, the circadian eating cycle is out of phase with the circadian sleep–wake cycle and causes one to consume excessive calories.

Night Terrors—a disorder of arousal associated with non-REM sleep initiated by a scream associated with panic, followed by intense autonomic activity such as sweating, rapid heart rate, and a terrified appearance. This is due to overactivity of the sympathetic fight-or-flight system. There can be associated motor activity resulting in injury due to running into walls or falling.

Nightmare Disorder—recurrent nightmares, generally in the REM sleep cycle, that are coherent dream sequences and manifest as disturbing mental experiences.

Nocturnal—takes place at night.

Nocturnal Groaning—disruptive groaning that occurs during expiration, particularly during the second half of night.

Non–Rapid Eye Movement Sleep (non-REM)—deep, dreamless sleep that occurs cyclically during a normal period of sleep and comprises three-fourths of the night's sleep, with intervening periods of REM sleep. Also termed non-REM sleep or slow-wave sleep comprised of sleep stages one, two, and slow-wave.

Obstructive Sleep Apnea (OSA) (Sleep Apnea Syndrome)—a sleep disorder where breathing is frequently interrupted for brief intervals during sleep, resulting in intermittent decreases in blood oxygen levels and transient arousals from sleep, leading to poor sleep quality and excessive daytime sleepiness.

Parasomnias—behaviors or experiences that occur during entry into sleep, during sleep, or during arousals from sleep. The behaviors include sleepwalking, sleep talking, and sleep terrors.

Periodic Limb Movements—rhythmic movement during sleep.

Photoperiod—the cycle of day and night or light and dark.

Photoreceptor—a molecule that detects light.

Polysomnogram—a sleep test that continuously acquires physiological data obtained during sleep, including brain wave activity, eye movements, muscle activity (chin and legs), heart rate, body position, and respiratory variables, including oxygen saturation.

Polysomnography—recording multiple bodily functions while a person sleeps.

Post-Traumatic Stress Disorder (PTSD)—a diagnosis of mental and emotional trauma after exposure to or experience of a trauma.

Rapid-Eye-Movement Sleep (REM)—deep sleep with rapid eye movements in which dreaming takes place.

REM Sleep Behavior Disorder (RSBD)—complex behaviors, including mild to harmful body movements associated with dreams and nightmares and loss of muscle atonia.

Restless Legs Syndrome (RLS)—a neurologic movement disorder that is often associated with a sleep complaint.

Seasonal Affective Disorder (SAD)—a form of depression caused by inadequate bright light.

Sexsomnia—when a person engages in sexual activities while asleep.

Shift Work Sleep Disorder—a circadian rhythm sleep disorder with insomnia and excessive sleepiness affecting people whose work hours are typically the night shift.

Sleep Apnea—a disorder of periodic stops in breathing during sleep caused by either an obstruction of the airway or a disturbance in the brain's breathing center.

Sleep Attacks—the sudden need or desire to go to sleep.

Sleep Deprivation—the disorder of not having adequate sleep.

Sleep Drunkenness—a problem in waking up and being confused for long periods of time after waking. Also known as sleep inertia.

Sleep Hygiene—the practice of maintaining proper sleep health.

Sleep Medicine—the medical specialty applied to the diagnosis and treatment of persons with chronic sleep loss or sleep disorders.

Sleep Paralysis—muscle paralysis akin to sleep atonia (REM sleep) while awake, when falling asleep, or waking up.

Sleep-Related Dissociative Disorder—dissociative episodes that can occur in the period from wakefulness to sleep or from awakening from stages 1 or 2 or from REM sleep.

Sleep-Related Eating Disorder (SRED)—repeated episodes of involuntary eating and drinking during arousals from sleep.

Sleep-Related Hallucination—hallucinatory images that occur at sleep onset or on awakening from sleep.

Sleep Restriction Therapy—a technique that restricts time in bed to the actual sleep time, which creates mild sleep deprivation and results in more efficient sleep.

Sleep Spindle—the hills and valleys of electrical brain activity at 7 to 14 Hz, grouped in sequences that last one to two seconds and recur periodically with a slow rhythm of 0.1 to 0.4 Hz.

Sleepwalking—a disorder of arousal in non-REM sleep involving a series of behaviors initiated during arousals from slow-wave sleep that culminate in walking around in an altered state of consciousness.

Slow-wave Sleep (SWS)—sleep stages characterized by slow waves.

Sleep Stages—sleep cycles in which different brain wave patterns are displayed.
- Stage 1—first stage of non-REM sleep characterized by low-voltage, mixed-frequency waves on the EEG; small, slow eye movements, and tonic muscles.
- Stage 2—cycle of non-REM sleep characterized by low-voltage, mixed-frequency waves on the EEG, sleep spindles, and K-complexes; occasional small eye movements near sleep onset; and tonic muscles.
- Stage 3—cycle of non-REM sleep characterized by high-voltage, slow-wave activity on the EEG; no eye movements; and tonic muscles.

Stimulus Control—technique to disrupt sleep, thus preventing associations with the bedroom by enhancing the likelihood of sleep.

Suprachiasmatic Nucleus (SCN)—the small area within the hypothalamus that contains the biological clock.

Thalamus—the area of the brain that relays sensory information to the cerebral cortex.

Ultradian Rhythm—a time period less than 24 hours.

Notes

Introduction

p. xvi: *Rather, we now know how active the sleeptime*: D. Markov and M. Goldman, "Normal Sleep and Circadian Rhythms: Neurobiological Mechanisms Underlying Sleep and Wakefulness," *Psychiatric Clinics of North America* 29, no. 4 (2006): 417.

Chapter 2

p. 9: *Most people experience*:   Ibid, 418.

p. 13: *In one study people deprived of sleep for a few days following an influenza vaccine*:   K. Spiegel, J. F. Sheridan, and E. Van Cauter, "Effect of Sleep Deprivation on Response to Immunization," *JAMA* 288, no. 12 (2002): 1471–72.

p. 13: *In one sleep study, researchers tested and examined the participants' specific levels of three inflammatory markers*:   Alanna Morris et al., "Sleep Quality and Duration Are Associated with Higher Levels of Inflammatory Biomarkers: The META-Health Study," *Circulation* 122 (2010): A17806.

p. 14: *If you sleep less than six hours per night*:   F. P. Cappuccio, D. Cooper, L. D'Elia, P. Strasullo, and M. A. Miller., "Sleep Duration Predicts Cardiovascular Outcomes: A Systematic Review and Meta-Analysis of Prospective Studies," *European Heart Journal* 32, no. 12 (2011): 1484–92.

p. 14: *A recent study revealed that cells that produce myelin*: M. Bellisi, M Pfister-Genskow, S. Maret, S. Keles, G. Tononi, and C. Cirelli, "Effects of Sleep and Wake on Oligodendrocytes and Their Precursors," *Journal of Neuroscience* 33, no. 36 (2013): 14288–300.

p. 14: *Another recent study of mice*: L. Xie *et al.*, "Sleep Drives Metabolite Clearance from the Adult Brain," *Science* 342, no. 6156 (2013): 373–77.

Chapter 4

p. 39: *one of the most prevalent neurological disorders*: K. Berger, J. Luedemann, C. Trenkwalder, U. John, and C. Kessler, "Sex and the Risk of Restless Legs Syndrome in the General Population," *Archives of Internal Medicine* 164 (2004): 196–202.

p. 40: *Women are more likely to suffer*: M. Viola-Saltman *et al.*, "High Prevalence of Restless Legs Syndrome among Patients with Fibromyalgia: A Controlled Cross-Sectional Study," *Journal of Clinical Sleep Medicine* 6, no. 5 (2010): 423–27.

p. 40: *Surveys have demonstrated*: J. Montplaisir, S. Boucher, G. Poirer, G. Lavigne, O. Lapierre, P. Lesperance, "Clinical, Polysomnographic, and Genetic Characteristics of Restless Legs Syndrome: A Study of 133 Patients Diagnosed with New Standard Criteria," *Movement Disorders* 12 (1997): 61–65.

p. 40: *Although commonly overlooked in children*: D. Picchietti *et al.*, "Restless Leg Syndrome: Prevalence and Impact in Children and Adolescents—the PEDS REST Study," *Pediatrics* 120, no. 2 (2007): 253–66.

p. 40: *Further evidence from the survey*: C. Trenkwalder, W. Paulus, and A. S. Walters. "The Restless Legs Syndrome," *Lancet Neurology* 4 (2005): 465–75.

p. 40: *Early onset is associated with increased severity*: S. Whittom, Y. Dauvilliers, M. H. Pennestri, F. Vercauteren, N. Molinari, and J. Montplasir, "Age-at-Onset in Restless

Legs Syndrome: A Clinical and Polysomnographic Study," *Sleep Medicine* 9, no. 1 (2007): 54–59. [Epub July 17, 2007].

p. 42: *Other effective treatments not involving medications*: U. H. Mitchell, "Non-Drug-Related Aspect of Treating Ekbom Disease, Formerly Known as Restless Legs Syndrome," *Neuropsychiatric Disease and Treatment* 7 (2011): 251–57.

p. 43: *In a recent study of laser therapy*: C. A. Hayes, J. R. Kingsley, K. R. Hamby, and J. Carlow, "The Effect of Endovenous Laser Ablation on Restless Legs Syndrome," *Phlebology* 23, no. 3 (2008): 112–17.

Chapter 5

p. 51: *Insomnia in younger adults*: C. M. Morin and S. E. Gramling, "Sleep Patterns and Aging: Comparison of Older Adults with and without Insomnia Complaints," *Psychology and Aging* 4 (1989): 290–94.

p. 55: *Another way to understand the development and continuance of primary insomnia*: A. J. Spielman, L. S. Caruso, and P. B. Glovinsky, "A Behavioral Perspective on Insomnia Treatment," *Psychiatric Clinics of North America* 10 (1987): 541–53.

p. 55: *I refer you to*: Elaine N. Aron, *The Highly Sensitive Person: How to Thrive When the World Overwhelms You* (New York: Birch Lane Press, 1996).

p. 64: *In fact, in one study of over 14,000 patients*: Ohayon MM, Roth T. "Place of Chronic Insomnia in the Course of Depressive and Anxiety Disorders." *Journal of Psychiatric Research* 37, no. 1 (2003): 9–15.

p. 64: *In addition, insomnia occurs*: Ibid.

p. 64: *A recent study from South Korea*: Jae-Huyn Kim, Eun-Cheoi Park, Woo-Hyn Cho, Chong Yon Park, Won-Jung Choi, and Hoo-Sun Chang, "Association Between Total Sleep Duration and Suicidal Ideation among the Korean General Adult Population," *Sleep* 36, no. 10 (2013): 1563–72.

p. 65: *underlying the dysfunctional emotion regulation*: P. Franzen, "Elevated Amygdala Activation During Voluntary Emotion Regulation in Primary Insomnia," *Sleep* (2013), accessed November 15, 2013, http://www.sciencedaily.com/releases/2013/05/130522131208.htm.

p. 67: *Women's research confirms*: M. Jepkema, "Insomnia," Health Reports, Statistics Canada, Catalogue 82-003, 17 (2005): 9–25.

p. 67: *The greatest news*: A. D. Krystal, "Treating the Health, Quality of Life, and Functional Impairments in Insomnia," *Journal of Clinical Sleep Medicine* 3, no. 1 (2007): 63–72.

p. 68: *Rise at a regular time every day*: C. M. Morin, "Cognitive-behavioral therapy of insomnia," *Sleep Medicine Clinics* 1 (2006): 375–86.

p. 70: *Seventy to eighty percent of people with insomnia*: D. F. Tolin, "Is Cognitive–Behavioral Therapy More Effective than Other Therapies? Meta-Analytic Review," *Clinical Psychology Review* 30, no. 6 (2010): 710–20.

p. 71: *In a book called:* Barry Krakow, *Sound Sleep, Sound Mind, 7 keys to Sleeping through the Night* (Hoboken, NJ: John Wiley & Sons, 2007).

Chapter 6

p. 85: *Other stimuli include*: T. Åkerstedt, "Sleepiness and Circadian Rhythm Sleep Disorders," *Sleep Medicine Clinics* 17 (2006): 17–30.

p. 85: *The function of these proteins*: Ibid, 421.

p. 86: *Melátonin affects the receptors in the SCN*: Ibid.

p. 87: *This is easily explained*: "Sleepy Connected Americans," *National Sleep Foundation Press Release* (March 7, 2011).

p. 89: *Studies show that east-to-west travel*: T. Åkerstedt, "Sleepiness and Circadian Rhythm Sleep Disorders," *Sleep Medicine Clinics* 23 (2006): 23–24.

p. 89: *Other symptoms include*: Ibid, 18.

p. 89: *There is also evidence to suggest*: Ibid, 23–24.

p. 89: *Symptoms checklist*: http://www.mayoclinic.com/ health/jetlag/DS01085/DSECTION=symptoms

p. 93: *They typically go to bed around the same time*: T. Åkerstedt, "Sleepiness and Circadian Rhythm Sleep Disorders," *Sleep Medicine Clinics* 23 (2006): 24.

p. 94: *Their melatonin and core body temperature*: L. C. Lack and H. R. Wright, "Clinical Management of Delayed Sleep Phase Disorder," *Behavioral Sleep Medicine* 5, no. 1 (2007): 58.

p. 94: *Some contend*: Ibid.

p. 96: *Characteristic of this disorder*: T. Åkerstedt, "Sleepiness and Circadian Rhythm Sleep Disorders," *Sleep Medicine Clinics* 23 (2006): 27.

p. 97: *About 50% of totally blind people*: R. L. Sack, "Circadian Rhythm Sleep Disorder: Part II, Adv-anced Sleep Phase Disorder, Delayed Sleep Phase Disorder, Free-Running Disorder, and Irregular Sleep–Wake Rhythm American Academy of Sleep Medicine," *Sleep* 30, no. 11 (2007–2008): 1492.

p. 97: *Others are able to structure*: Ibid.

p. 98: *Most of the people with this disorder are elderly*: T. Åkerstedt, "Sleepiness and Circadian Rhythm Sleep Disorders," *Sleep Medicine Clinics* 23 (2006): 27.

p. 100: *report difficulty falling asleep:* American Psychiatric Publishing, *Diagnostic and Statistical Manual of Mental Disorders*, 4th ed., text revision (Washington, DC: American Psychiatric Association, 2000).

p. 100: *Self-assessment surveys show*: Ibid, 22.

p. 100: *As a result, shift work sleep disorder*: Ibid, 21.

p. 101: *Bright light treatment*: C. I. Eastman, K. T. Stewart, M. P. Mahoney, L. Liu, and L. F. Fogg, "Dark Goggles and Bright Light Improve Circadian Rhythm Adaptation to Night-Shift Work," *Sleep* 17, no. 6 (1994): 535–43.

p. 101: *This disorder is also treated with melatonin*: R. L. Sack and A. J. Lewy, "Melatonin as a Chronobiotic: Treatment of Circadian Desynchrony in Night Workers and the Blind," *Journal of Biological Rhythms* 12, no. 6 (1997):595.

p. 108: *Self-Assessment for Night Owls and Morning Larks*: Adapted from J. A. Horne and O. Östberg, "A Self-Assessment Questionnaire to Determine Morningness–Eveningness in Human Circadian Rhythms," *International Journal Chronobiology* 4, no. 2 (1976): 97–110.

Chapter 7

p. 112–13: *Both pilots unintentionally fell asleep*: L. Ferini-Strambi C. Baietto, M. R. Di Gioia, P. Castaldi, C. Castronovo, M. Zucconi, and S. F. Cappa, "Cognitive Dysfunction in Patients with Obstructive Sleep Apnea (OSA): Partial Reversibility after Continuous Positive Airway Pressure (CPAP)," *Brain Research Bulletin* 61 (2003): 87–92.

p. 113: *driver's fatigue, caused by the combined effects*: "Tractor Semitrailer Rear-End Collision into Passenger Vehicles on Interstate 44 near Miami, Oklahoma, June 26, 2009." *Highway Accident Report.* Washington DC: National Transportation Safety Board. Report NTSB/HAR-10/02.

p. 113: *failure of the crew*: M. R. Rosekind, "*The Role of Sleep Loss in Transportation Accidents: NTSB Investigations and Recommendation.*" National Transportation Safety Board presentation at UPenn School of Medicine (February 20, 2013).

p. 113: *A recent study showed*: Nathaniel S. Marshall, Keith K. H. Wong, Peter Y. Liu, Stewart R. J. Cullen, Matthew W. Knuiman, and Ronald R. Grunstein, "Sleep apnea as an independent risk factor for all-cause mortality: The Busselton Health Study," *Sleep* 31, no. 8 (2008): 1079–85.

p. 114: *Obstructive Sleep Apnea is a common disorder*: Adult Obstructive Sleep Apnea Task Force of the American Academy of Sleep Medicine, "Guideline for Evaluation, Management, and Long-Term Care of Obstructive Sleep Apnea in Adults," *Journal of Clinical Sleep Medicine* 5, no. 3 (2009): 263–76.

p. 117: *In part, because of this, recent studies:* David W. Hudgel, Lois E. Lamerato, Gordon R. Jacobsen, and

Christopher L. Drake, "Assessment of multiple health risks in a single obstructive sleep apnea population,"*Journal of Clinical Sleep Medicine* 15, no. 8 (2012): 9–18.

p. 118: *A study presented at the 2013 American Thoracic Society International Conference*: Sushmita Pamidi Magddalena Stepien, Khalid Sharif-Sidi, Harry Whitmore, Lisa Morselli, Kristen Wroblewski, and Ersa Tasali, "Effective Treatment of Obstructive Sleep Apnea Improves Glucose Tolerance in Prediabetes: A Randomized, Placebo-Controlled Trial," *American Thoracic Society Meeting* (May 20, 2013). Available at www.atsjournals.org/doi/abs/10.1164/ajrccm-conference.2013.187.1_MeetingAbstracts.A2381

p. 121: *Definitely, sleep apnea relates to erectile dysfunction*: Stephan Budweiser, Stefan Enderlein, Rudolf A Jörres, Andre P. Hitzl, Wolf F. Wieland, Michael Pfeifer, and Michael Arzt, "Sleep Apnea Is an Independent Correlate of Erectile and Sexual Dysfunction," *Journal of Sexual Medicine* 6, no. 11 (2009): 3147–57.

p. 122: *The prevalence of men*: A. D. Seftel *et al.*, "Erectile Dysfunction and Symptoms of Sleep Disorders," *Sleep* 25 (2002): 643–47.

p. 122: *In fact, studies have shown*: Francesco Fanfulla, Antonio Camera, Paola Fulgoni, Luca Chiovato, and Rossella E. Nappi, "Sexual dysfunction in obese women: does obstructive sleep apnea play a role?" *Sleep Medicine* 14, no. 3 (2013): 252–56.

Chapter 8

p. 129: *Another recent study showed*: E. Yilmaz, K. Sedky, and D. S. Bennettet, "The Relationship between Depressive Symptoms and Obstructive Sleep Apnea in Pediatric Populations: A Meta-Analysis," *Journal of Clinical Sleep Medicine* 9, no. 11 (2013): 1213–20.

p. 138: *Sleepwalking is more prevalent*: G. Stores. "Parasomnias of Childhood and Adolescence," *Sleep Medicine Clinics* 2 (2007): 405–17.

p. 139: *Treatment effects were maintained*: N. C. Frank *et al.*, "The Use of Scheduled Awakenings to Eliminate

Childhood Sleepwalking," *Journal of Pediatric Psychology* 22, no. 3 (1997): 345–53.

p. 139: *According to a 2012 study*: M. M. Ohayon *et al.*, "Prevalence and Comorbidity of Nocturnal Wandering in the US Adult General Population," *Neurology* 78, no. 20 (2012): 1583–89.

p. 140: *One cohort research project*: Jacques Montplasir, Dominique Petit, Mathieu Pilon, Valerie Mongrain, and Antonio Zadra, "Does Sleepwalking Impair Daytime Vigilance?" *Journal of Clinical Sleep Medicine* 7 (2011): 219.

p. 140: *The pattern of inheritance*: A. K. Licis, D. M. Desruisseau, K. A. Yamada, S. P. Duntley, and C. A. Gurnett, "Novel Genetic Findings in an Extended Family Pedigree with Sleepwalking," *Neurology* 76, no. 1 (2011): 49–52.

p. 140: *They determined that sleepwalking*: Ibid.

Chapter 9

p. 146: *Two doctors, Schenck and Mahowald*: C. H. Schenck, I. Arnulf, and M. W. Mahowald, "Sleep and Sex: What Can Go Wrong? A Review of the Literature on Sleep-Related Disorders and Abnormal Sexual Behaviors and Experiences," *Sleep* 30, no. 6 (2007): 683–702.

p. 147: *she did believe her husband's accounts*: Antonio Culebras, *Case Studies in Sleep Neurology, Common and Uncom-mon Presentations* (United Kingdom: Cambridge University Press, 2010), 33.

p. 148: *The official list of sexsomnia behaviors*: P. R. Buchanan. "Sleep Sex," *Sleep Medicine Clinics* 6, no. 4 (2011): 417–28.

p. 152: *A recent study from Stanford*: C. Guilleminault, "Sexual Behaviors during Sleep," *Stanford Journal of Sleep Epidemiology* V (2011): 1.

p. 153: *Somnambulism or sleepwalking is a viable defence*: E. I. Osman, "Somnambulistic Sexual Behaviour (Sexsomnia)," *Journal of Clinical Forensic Medicine* 13, no. 4 (2006): 219–24.

Chapter 10

p. 156: *They are also indicative*: J. B. Zawilska, E. J. Santorek-Strumiłło, and P. Kuna, "Nighttime Eating

Disorders: Clinical Symptoms and Treatment," *Przeglad Lekarski* 67, no. 7 (2010): 536–40 (Polish).

p. 158: *These episodes have been described*: L. M. Howell, C. Schenck, and S. J. Crow, "Curbing Nocturnal Binges in Sleep-Related Eating Disorder," *Current Psychiatry* 6, no. 7 (2007): 21.

p. 161: *Between 30% and 50% of their daily caloric*: Cristoph J. Lauer and Jürgen-Christian Krieg, "Sleep in Eating Disorders," *Sleep Medicine Review* 8 , no. 2 (2004): 109.

p. 161: *However, unlike SRED*: Ibid.

p. 162: *For a definitive diagnosis*: L. M. Howell, C. Schenck, and S. J. Crow, "Curbing Nocturnal Binges in Sleep-Related Eating Disorder," *Current Psychiatry* 6, no. 7 (2007): 21.

p. 162: *Given NES's co-morbidity*: Ibid.

p. 163: *Cognitive behavioral therapy was first used*: K. C. Allison and E. P. Tarves, "Treatment of Night Eating Syndrome," *Psychiatric Clinics of North America* 34, no. 4 (2011): 785–96.

Chapter 11

p. 169: *Violent episodes typically happen:* American Academy of Sleep Medicine. *International Classification of Sleep Disorders, Revised: Diagnostic and Coding Manual* (Chicago: American Academy of Sleep Medicine, 2001), 97.

p. 170: *REM refers to*: M. A. Carskadon, W. C. Dement, "Normal Human Sleep: An Overview," in *Monitoring and Staging Human Sleep*, ed. M. H. Kryger, T. Roth, and W. C. Dement, *Principles and Practice of Sleep Medicine*, 5th ed. (St. Louis: Elsevier Saunders, 2011), 16–26.

p. 173: *New evidence establishes RSBD*: B. F. Boeve et al., "Clinicopathologic Correlations in 172 Cases of Rapid Eye Movement Sleep Behavior Disorder with or vwithout a Coexisting Neurologic Disorder," *Sleep Medicine* 14, no. 8 (2013): 754–62, doi:10.1016/j.sleep.2012.10.015.

Chapter 12

p. 184: *The estimated rate of lifetime*: "A Supplemental Take-Home Module for the NAMI Family-to-Family Education Program: Understanding and Coping with PTSD,"

Veterans Healthcare Administration, National Center for PTSD (Updated, January, 2011), accessed November 25, 2011, www.ncptsd.va.gov.

p. 184: *Children's trauma*: B. A. van der Kolk. "Developmental Trauma Disorder: Towards a Rational Diagnosis for Children with Complex Trauma Histories," Pre-publication version. accessed November 15, 2013, http://traumacenter.org.

p. 185: *An estimated one out of nine*: Ibid.

p. 186: *That 70% to 91% of patients*: M. J. Maker, S. A. Rego, and G. M. Asnis, "Sleep Disturbances in Patients with Post-Traumatic Stress Disorder," *CNS Drugs* 20, no. 7 (2006): 567–90.

p. 186: *A research review correlated*: P. Gillar, M. Atul, and L. Peretz, "Post-Traumatic Stress Disorder and Sleep— What a Nightmare!" *Sleep Medicine Reviews* 4, no. 2 (2000): 183–200.

p. 188: *This provided further possibility*: D. Collen et al., "Sleep Disorders in Operation Iraqi Freedom and Operation Enduring Freedom Veterans," *Meeting Abstratcs* 140, no. 4 (2011): 567–73.

p. 189: *The hippocampus checks*: L. Baird, "Childhood Trauma in the Etiology of Borderline Personality Disorder: Theoretical Considerations and Therapeutic Interventions," *Hakomi Forum*, Issue 19-20-21 (2008): 31–42.

p. 190: *Sleep apnea may*: "Post-Traumatic Stress Disorder," *New York Times, Health Guide*, http://www.nytimes.com/health/guides/disease/post-traumatic-stress-disorder/print.html

p. 190: *Treating sleep apnea*: Press release: "CPAP Therapy Reduces Nightmares in Veterans with PTSD and Sleep Apnea," *American Academy of Sleep Medicine.* Accessed November 15, 2013, http://www.aasmnet.org/articles.aspx?id=4032

p. 190: *The first large-scale study*: A. D. Seelig, I. G. Jacobson, B.Smith, T. I. Hooper, E. J. Boyko, G. D. Gackstetter,

P. Gehrman, C. A. Macera, T. C. Smith, Millennium Cohort Study Team, "Sleep Patterns Before, During, and After Deployment to Iraq and Afghanistan," *Sleep* 33, no. 12 (2012): 1615–22.

p. 191: *According to the study*: P. Gehrman, A. D. Seelig, I. G. Jacobsen, E. J. Boyko, T. I. Hooper, G. D. Gackstetter, C. S. Ulmer, and T. C. Smith, "Predeployment Sleep Duration and Insomnia Symptoms as Risk Factors for New-Onset Mental Health Disorders Following Military Deployment," *Sleep* 36, no. 7 (2013): 1009–18.

p. 192: *Treating insomnia and other sleep disorder*: A. Germain, "Sleep-Specific Mechanisms Underlying Post-Traumatic Stress Disorder: Integrative Review and Neurobiological Hypotheses," *Sleep Medicine Reviews* 12, no. 3 (2008): 185–95.

Chapter 13

p. 198: *The estimated percentage*: E. G. Willcutt, "The Prevalence of *DSM-IV* Attention-Deficit\Hyperactivity Disorder: A Meta-Analytic Review," *Neurotherapeutics* 9, no. 93 (July 2012): 490–99.

p. 198: *A long-term study following young children*: Ibid.

p. 199: *One sleep study*: S. Shur-Fen Gau, "Prevalence of Sleep Problems and Their Association with Inattention/ Hyperactivity among Children Aged 6–15 in Taiwan," *Journal of Sleep Research* 15, no. 4 (2006): 403–14.

p. 199: *As a result of being sleepy*: S. Shur-Fen Gau, "Prevalence of Sleep Problems and Their Association with Inattention/Hyperactivity Among Children Aged 6–15 in Taiwan," *Journal of Sleep Research* 15, no. 4 (2006):403–14.

p. 199: *In a study reported in the* British Journal of Epidemiology: Y. Kelly, J. Kelly, and A. Sacker, "Time for Bed: Associations with Cognitive Performance in 7-Year-Old Children: A Longitudinal Population-Based Study," *Journal of Epidemiology and Community Health* 67 (2013): 202–04. doi:10.1136/jech-2012. 202024.

p. 199: *The authors concluded*: Y. Kelly, J. Kelly, and A. Sacker, "Changes in Bedtime Schedules and Behavioral Difficulties in 7-Year-Old Children," *Pediatrics* 14 (2013). doi: 10.1542/peds.2013–1906.

p. 200: *A more recent study published in the* Journal of Pediatric Psychology: J. L. Vriend, F. D, Davidson, P. V. Corkum, C. T. Chambers, and E, N. McLaughlin, "Manipulating Sleep Duration Alters Emotional Functioning and Cognitive Performance in Children," *Journal of Pediatric Psychology* 38, no. 10 (2013): 1058–69.

p. 201: *A recently published comprehensive study*: N. Scott, P. S. Blair, A. M. Emond, P. J. Fleming, J. S. Humphreys, J. Henderson, and P. Gringras, "Sleep Patterns in Children with ADHD: A Population-Based Cohort Study from Birth to 11 Years," *Journal of Sleep Research* 2, (2013): 121–28.

p. 201: *In a vicious cycle*: A. Prehn-Kristensen, M. Munz, I. Molzow, I. Wilhem, C. D. Wiesner, and L. Baving, "Sleep Promotes Consolidation of Emotional Memory in Healthy Children but Not in Children with Attention-Deficit Hyperactivity Disorder," *PLOS ONE* 8, no. 5 (2013): e65098, doi:10.1371/journal.pone.0065098

p. 202: *After treatment for the sleep apnea*: N. A. Youssef, M. Ege, S. S. Angly, J. L. Strauss, and C. E. Marx, "Is Obstructive Sleep Apnea Associated with ADHD?" *Annals of Clinical Psychiatry* 23, no. 3 (2011): 213–24.

p. 202: *Many with ADD*: T. E. Brown, "AD/HD and Co-Occurring Conditions," *Attention Magazine* (February 2009): 10–15.

p. 203: *A cross-sectional survey*: R. D. Chervin, K. H. Archbold, J. E. Dillon, K. J. Pituch, P. Panahi, R. E. Dahl, and C. Guilleminault, "Associations Between Symptoms of Inattention, Hyperactivity, Restless Legs, and Periodic Leg Movements," *Journal of Sleep Research and Sleep Medicine* 25, no. 2 (2002): 213–18.

p. 203: *Children with ADHD have an increased*: D. L. Picchietti, S. J. England, A. S. Walters, K. Willis, and T. Verrico, "Periodic Limb Movement Disorder and Restless Legs Syndrome in Children with Attention-Deficit

Hyperactivity Disorder," *Journal of Child Neurology* 13, no. 12 (1980): 588–94.

p. 203: *Children with periodic limb movement*: D. L. Picchietti, "Further Studies on Periodic Limb Movement Disorder and Restless Legs Syndrome in Children with Attention-Deficit Hyperactivity Disorder," *Movement Disorders* 14, no. 6 (1999): 1000–07.

p. 203: *Treatment of PLM*: A. S. Walters, D. E. Mandelbaum, D. S. Lewis, S. Kugler, S. J. England, and M. Miller, "Dopaminergic Therapy in Children with Restless Legs/ Periodic Limb Movements in Sleep and ADHD. Dopaminergic Therapy Study Group," *Pediatric Neurology* 22, no. 1 (2000): 82–86.

p. 204: *Three to twelve percent of children have incidents*: E. Hulcrantz, B. Lofstarnd-Tideström, and J. Ahlquist-Rastad "The Epidemiology of Sleep Related Breathing Disorders in Children. *International Journal of Pediatric Otorhinolaryngology*, 32, Suppl. (1995): S63–S66.

p. 204: *The good news is*: R. D. Chervin, D. L. Ruzicka, B. J. Giordani, R. A. Weatherly, J. E. Dillon, E. K. Hodges, C. L. Marcus, and K. E. Guire, "Sleep-Disordered Breathing, Behavior, and Cognition in Children Before and After Adenotonsillectomy," *Pediatrics* 117 (2006): e769–e778.

p. 204: *A recent NIH-sponsored study*: C. L. Marcus, "A Randomized Trial of Adenotonsillectomy for Childhood Sleep Apnea," *New England Journal of Medicine* 368 (2013): 2366–76.

p. 207: *In one study, researchers compared*: M. Osterloo, G. J. Lammers, S. Overeem, I. de Noord, and J. J. Kooij, "Possible Confusion Between Primary Hypersomnia and Adult Attention-Deficit/Hyperactivity Disorder," *Psychiatry Research* 143, no. 2–3 (2006): 293–97 [Epub July 18, 2006].

p. 208: *One study concluded that*: M. L. Wagner, A. S. Walters, and B. C. Fisher, "Symptoms of Attention-Deficit/

Hyperactivity Disorder in Adults with Restless Legs Syndrome," *American Academy of Sleep Medicine* 27, no. 8 (2004): 1499–504.

p. 208: *As compared with control groups*:   A. L. Baird, "Adult Attention-Deficit Hyperactivity Disorder is Associated with Alterations in Circadian Rhythms at the Behavioural, Endocrine and Molecular Levels," *Molecular Psychiatry* 17, no. 10 (2012): 988–95.

Acknowledgments

I would like to extend a heartfelt thank you to my amazing publicist Steve Allen from Steve Allen Media and Devra Jacobs, my incredible book agent from Dancing Word Group, for their guidance and support. To my editors Dr. Caron Goode and Susan Sparling-Micks, whose talents I admire. Lastly, to Julia Pastore from Demos Health Publishing, thank you for believing in sleep medicine and me.

Index

acetylcholine, 25
acid reflux, 46
actigraphs, 200
acute adjustment insomnia,
    51, 58–60
acute trauma, 184
adaptation, 19–20
Adaptive Servo Ventilator,
    127, 132, 133
adrenaline, 14, 25
advanced sleep-phase syndrome
    (ASPS), 96, 107–110
aging, 107
airline accidents, 112
alarm clocks, 22, 56
alcohol, 25, 42, 54, 67, 115,
    218–219
allergies, 13
alpha waves, 10
Alzheimer's disease, 14, 102
Ambien, 75, 144, 156, 158, 165
American Academy of Sleep
    Medicine, 75
amygdala, 189
anti-anxiety antidepressant
    medications, 63
antidepressant medications, 63, 75

antidepressants, 44, 175
antihistamines, 74
anxiety, 22, 27–28, 60–61, 68, 219
anxiety disorders, 40, 63, 190
arousal parasomnias, 135
asthma, 13
atherosclerosis, 13
atrial fibrillation, 115
atrial natriuretic peptide, 121
attention deficit hyperactivity
    disorder (ADHD), 198–211
  in adolescents, 207–209
  in adults, 207–209
  checklist, 221
  in children, 198–208
  daytime sleepiness and,
    202, 211
  defined, xx
  diagnosis of, 201
  prevalence of, 198
  restless legs syndrome and, 40,
    47, 202–203
  sleep apnea and, 120, 210
  sleep disorders associated with,
    202–208
  symptoms of, 198
  treatment for, 209

atypical antipsychotics, 194–195
augmentation, 46
autonomic nervous system,
    117–118

baths, 25
bedroom environment, 21–24, 217
bedroom rituals, 68
bedtime rituals, 55–56, 213,
    219–220
Benadryl, 42
benzodiazepines, 175
beta amyloid, 15
beta-blockers, 74, 175
beta waves, 10
bipolar disorder, 143, 164
blood pressure, 14, 117
blood sugar, 130
blue color, 22
blue light, 21, 24, 26, 86–88
blue light blocker glasses,
    87–88
body temperature, 25
brain
    PTSD and, 189–190
    sleep apnea and, 117–118, 123
brain dump, 28
brain fog, 15–18
brainwaves, 9, 10–11
bulimia, 157

caffeine, 25, 42, 54, 56, 77,
    80, 218
car accidents, 112, 113
carbidopa-levodopa, 46
carbon dioxide, 126–127
cardiovascular disease, 14
CBT. *See* cognitive behavioral
    therapy
central sleep apnea (CSA), 111,
    125–127, 128
Cheyne-Stokes breathing, 126
Childhood Adenotonsillectomy
    Trial (CHAT), 204
childhood obesity, 12

children
    with ADHD, 198–208
    checklist for, 205–207
    night terrors in, 142
    restless legs syndrome in, 40
    self-check for, 211
    sleep apnea and, 119,
        128–129, 201
    sleep needs of, 199–200
    sleepwalking in, 138–139
    trauma experienced by, 184
chronic inflammation, 13
chronic insomnia, 63–65, 76
chronic stress, 185
cigarettes, 24, 78
circadian biology, 84–88
circadian clock, 25, 68, 84–86,
    103–104
circadian rhythm disorders,
    84–110
    advanced sleep-phase
        syndrome, 96, 107–110
    defined, xix
    delayed sleep-phase syndrome,
        93–96, 107–110
    free-running disorder, 96–97
    irregular sleep–wake syndrome,
        98–99
    jet lag disorder, 88–93, 103
    questions about, 101–107
    self-check, 107–110
    shift work sleep disorder,
        99–101, 103–104
citalopram (Celexa), 166
clonazepam, 154, 160, 168, 175, 177
clutter, 23
coffee, 77
cognitive behavioral therapy
    (CBT), 57, 69–70, 163, 183,
    193, 197
cognitive development, 171,
    199–200
cognitive dysfunction, 13
cognitive restructuring, 56–57, 62,
    69–70

compact fluorescent lighting
(CFL) bulbs, 87
complex sleep apnea, 127,
132, 133
constructive worrying, 28
continuous positive airway
pressure (CPAP), 118,
123–124, 130–133
coping skills, 78
cortisol, 22, 65, 208, 218
C-reactive protein, 13

daytime sleepiness, 1, 13,
120, 211
declarative memory, 211
delayed sleep phase syndrome
(DSPS), 93–96, 102–103,
107–110
delta waves, 9, 11
dementia, sleep apnea and, 129
depression, 40, 64
developmental trauma, 184
diabetes, 13, 118–119, 130
diphenhydramine, 42, 210
dopamine, 40, 41, 46, 160
dopamine agonists, 203
doxylamine, 42
dreaming, 170, 172–173
dreams
acting out in, 176
violent, 175–176
driving, while asleep, 144
dyssomnias, 35
circadian rhythm disorders,
84–110
insomnia, 51–83
restless legs syndrome, 36–50
sleep apnea, 111–134
types of, xix

early morning awakenings, 62
electronic devices, 24, 56, 217,
87–88
emotional tension, releasing,
72–74

endocrine system, 118
endothelial dysfunction, 121
epilepsy, 131
erectile dysfunction (ED), 121
estrogen, 122
eszopiclone (Lunesta), 75
exercise, 42, 219
restless legs syndrome and, 48

fatigue, 15–18
feet, rubbing together, 45–46
female sexual dysfunction
(FSD), 122
ferritin, 41, 141, 210
fibrinogen, 13
fibromyalgia, 39, 48
fight-or-flight response, 118
flurazepam (Dalmane), 74
f.Lux, 88
fog brain, 15–18
foot pain, 44
forgetfulness, 16
free radicals, 122
free-running disorder, 96–97

GABA (gamma-aminobutyric
acid), 74
gambling addiction, 45
General Anxiety Score (GAD-7), 61
ghrelin, 12
glucose, 155
green color, 23
guided imagery, 73

habits
to aid sleep, 25–26
that interfere with sleep,
24–25, 61
health
impact of sleep deprivation on,
12–15, 105–106
importance of sleep to, 8
heartburn, 13
hippocampus, 87, 189
histamine, 74

Horne–Ostberg test, 107
hot flashes, 67
hyperarousal, 55–56, 58, 66, 187
hyperarousal syndrome, 73
hyperphagia, 161
hypertension, 14, 115
hypoglossal nerve stimulator
    (HPNS), 124
hypopnea, 111

imagery rehearsal therapy, 183,
    193, 197
immune system, 13, 105
incandescent light bulbs, 87
inflammation, 13–14
inflammatory conditions, 13
inflammatory mediators, 119
insomnia, 51–83
    causes of, 65–66
    chronic, 63–65, 76
    defined, xix
    denial of, 78–79
    depression and, 64
    with multiple causal factors,
        60–63
    prevalence of, 51
    primary, 52–58
    psychophysiological, 54–55
    PTSD and, 186, 190–192, 196
    questions about, 76–82
    self-check, 83
    sleep maintenance, 76
    symptoms of, 57–58
    transient, 51, 58–60
    treatment for, 56–58, 67–74, 79
    vulnerability to, 66–67
    women and, 66–67
Insomnia Severity Index (ISI), 83
insulin, 155
insulin resistance, 13, 130
interleukin-6, 13
iron, 41, 42, 141, 210
irregular sleep–wake syndrome,
    98–99
irregulary sleep wake disorder, 102

jet lag disorder, 88–93, 103
    symptoms, 89
    treatment for, 90–93
journals, 73

larks, 96
laser ablation, 42
leptin, 12
leukotriene inhibitors, 81
light box, 163
light bulbs, 24, 87
light-emitting diode (LED)
    bulbs, 87
lighting, 21, 24, 85, 86–88, 101
light therapy, 100, 104
limbic system, 118, 123
lithium, 143

magnesium, 42
mandibular advancement device
    (MAD), 124
medications. *See also specific types*
    for ADHD, 209–210
    antidepressants, 62, 75, 175
    pain, 126
    for PTSD, 193–196, 197
    RLS and, 46–47
    for RSBD, 175
    for sexsomnia, 154
    sleep, 74–75, 79
    to stay awake, 106
melanopsin, 86
melatonin, 24, 74, 85, 86–87, 95,
    106, 175, 176, 209
memory problems, 130
menopause, 67
menses, 67
mental ruminations, 22
men with sleep apnea, 121
methadone, 133–134
metoclopramide, 46
Millennium Cohort
    Study, 191
Mirapex, 47
Modafinil, 101

mood disorders, 120
morning anorexia, 161
morning light therapy, 95
motivation, identifying your,
    19–20
multiple sclerosis, 14
myelin, 14

naps, 218, 16
National Sleep Foundation, 12
natural disasters, 184
near-death experiences, 184
neurological disease, 173, 175
neuropathy, 42, 44
nicotine, 24, 42, 78, 218–219
night eating disorders, 155–166
    defined, xx
    incidence of, 156
    nocturnal eating syndrome, 156,
        160–164, 166
    questions about, 164–165
    self-check, 166
    sleep-related eating disorder,
        156–160, 163
    types of, 156
nightmares, 186, 192, 194–197
night owls, 93
night terrors, 137, 142–143
nighttime urination, 121
nocturnal eating syndrome (NES),
    155, 156, 160–164, 166
nonbenzodiazepines, 75
non-rapid eye movement (REM)
    parasomnias, 135
non-REM sleep, 9
noradrenaline, 14, 25, 65
norepinephrine, 173, 186, 196
noticing, 72
Nuvigil, 106
NyQuil, 42

obesity, 12, 124
obsession, 45
obsessive-compulsive
    disorder, 190

obstructive sleep apnea (OSA),
    111, 114–125
    brain and, 117–118
    in children, 119, 201, 203–205
    vs. CSA, 127
    diabetes and, 118–119
    factors contributing to,
        114–115
    hypertension and,
        115–117
    self-check, 134
    stroke and, 115–117
    symptoms of, 114, 120–123
    treatment of, 122–124
online CBT, 71
orexin, 79
over-the-counter sleep aids,
    74, 79
oxidative stress, 122

pain medications, 126
panic disorder, 190
PAP-NAP, 124
paradoxical sleep, 76–77
parasomnias, 135–136
    arousal, 135
    night eating disorders,
        155–166
    night terrors, 137, 142–143
    REM, 135
    REM sleep behavior disorder,
        167–178
    sexsomnia, 146–154
    sleepwalking, 137–142
    types of, xix–xx
parasympathetic nervous
    system, 117
Parkinson's disease, 173, 176
perimenopause, 67
period genes, 85–86
periodic leg movements, 141
periodic limb movement (PLM),
    43, 62, 203
perpetuating behaviors for
    insomnia, 55

Per protein, 85–86
pets, 22
pineal gland, 86
pneumatic compression, 42
Positive Airway Pressure Nap
    (PAP-NAP), 124
post-traumatic stress disorder
    (PTSD), 180–197
  case study of, 180–183
  checklist, 187
  defined, xx, 183–187
  insomnia and, 190–192, 196
  medications for, 195, 197
  nightmares and, 192, 194–197
  night terrors and, 143
  questions about, 193–197
  sleep apnea and, 189–190,
    193, 194
  sleep disorders related to,
    188–189
  symptoms of, 185–187
  treatment for, 192–193
  types of trauma triggering,
    184–185
  veterans with, 123
potassium, 42
pramipexole (Mirapex), 141,
    160, 176
prazosin, 190, 193, 194, 196, 197
precipitating events for
    insomnia, 55
prediabetes, 118, 130
predispositions to insomnia, 55
primary CSA, 126
primary insomnia, 52–58
progesterone, 122
progressive muscle relaxation,
    28–30, 73
Provigil, 106
psychological theory of insomnia,
    65
psychophysiological insomnia,
    54–55
PTSD. *See* post-traumatic stress
    disorder

rapid eye movement (REM) sleep,
    9–10, 11, 118
red light, 21, 87
relaxation, 72–74
REM parasomnias, 135–136
REM sleep. *See* rapid eye
    movement (REM) sleep
REM sleep behavior disorder
    (RSBD), 167–178
  about, 167–168
  defined, xx
  medications for, 175
  questions about, 175–178
  symptoms of, 169–170
  treatment of, 174–175
Requip, 45
restless legs syndrome (RLS), 36–50
  ADHD and, 47, 202–203
  antidepressants and, 44
  case study of, 36–39
  causes of, 410, 210
  defined, xix, 39–41
  diagnostic criteria for, 38–39
  exercise and, 48
  fibromyalgia and, 48
  genetic component of, 40
  medications and, 46–47
  nonpharmacological treatments
    for, 48
  obsession and, 45
  vs. periodic limb movements, 43
  prevalence of, 39
  primary, 39
  questions about, 43–49
  secondary, 39
  self-check, 49–50
  sleep attacks and, 47
  symptoms of, 36–39, 41
  treatment for, 41–43
  varicose veins and, 49–50
retinal ganglion cells, 86
reverse first night effects, 68
Ritalin, 47
RLS. *See* restless legs syndrome
room color, 22–23

room temperature, 21, 217
RSBD. *See* REM sleep behavior
    disorder

SAD lamps, 102–103
scheduled awakenings, 138
sclerotherapy, 42, 49
secondary CSA, 126
Seroquel, 194–195
serotonin, 163, 173
sertraline (Zoloft), 163, 166,
    195–196
sexsomnia, 146–154
    behaviors, 147–149
    causes of, 149
    as defense, 152–153
    defined, xix
    medications for, 154
    questions about, 154
    treatment for, 149–152
sexual dysfunction, 121–122
shift workers, 26, 86, 88, 105–107
shift work sleep disorder, 99–101,
    103–104
Sinemet, 46
Singulair, 81
sleep
    as active neurobiological state,
      xviii
    best practices for, 217–220
    as cornerstone of health, 8
    habits that interfere with,
      24–25, 61
    habits to aid, 25, 212–214
    importance of, xvii, 8
    non-REM, 9
    REM, 9–11, 118
    stages of, 9
sleep aids, 104
sleep apnea, 22, 111–134
    about, 111
    accidents caused by, 112–113
    ADHD and, 203–205, 210
    blood sugar and, 130
    brain and, 117–118, 123

    central, 125–127, 128
    in children, 119, 128–129, 201,
      203–205, 207
    complex, 127, 132, 133
    defined, xix
    dementia and, 129
    diabetes and, 118–119
    diagnosis of, 122
    epilsepsy, 131
    health risks of, 113
    obstructive, 114–125
    prevalence of, 113, 193
    PTSD and, 189–190, 193, 194
    questions about, 127–133
    self-check, 134
    stroke and, 115–117
    symptoms of, 111–112, 114,
      120–123
    treatment of, 122–124
sleep attacks, 47
sleep clinics, 122
sleep cycles, 9–12
sleep debt, 77
sleep deprivation
    chronic, 77
    effects of, xviii, 8, 12–18
    illness and, 105–106
    sleepwalking and, 139
sleep diary, 30–34
Sleep Disorder Checklist, 3–6
sleep disordered breathing,
    203–205
sleep disorders
    ADHD and, 198–211
    dyssomnias, 35
      circadian rhythm disorders,
        84–110
      insomnia, 51–83
      restless legs syndrome, 36–50
      sleep apnea, 111–134
    identifying, 1–6
    parasomnias, 135–136
      night eating disorders,
        155–166
      night terrors, 137, 142–143

REM sleep behavior disorder,
167–178
sexsomnia, 146–154
sleepwalking, 137–142
prevalence of, xx
PTSD and, 180
sleep driving, 144
sleep environment, 217
sleep hygiene, 56, 61, 67, 209, 212
sleep inertia, 101
sleepiness
daytime, 1, 13, 120, 211
melatonin and, 86
sleeping environment, 21–24
sleep maintenance insomnia, 76
sleep medications, 74–75, 79
sleep-preventing behaviors, 55
sleep-related eating disorder
(SRED), 156–160, 163
sleep restriction, 69, 79–80
sleep routine, 217–218
sleep specialists, preparation for
appointment with, 75–76
sleep studies, 63, 194
sleep time
decrease in, xviii
inadequate, 8, 12
sleep–wake cycle, 68, 96, 98, 103
sleepwalking, 137–142
in adults, 139–142, 144
in children, 138–139
defined, xix
genetic component of, 140, 144
lithium and, 143
questions about, 143–145
treatment for, 138
triggers, 140
slow wave sleep, 9
smoking, 78
snoring, 22, 111–112, 203–204
somnambulism, 137–142
sound, 21–22
stage 1 sleep, 9
stimuli, 85
stimulus control, 56, 62, 68–69

stress, 72, 77–78, 154, 185
stress hormones, 14, 22, 25,
65, 118
stroke, 115
sugar, 164
suicidal ideation, 64
sunlight, 25
suprachiasmatic nucleus (SCN),
85–86
sympathetic nervous system,
117–118, 189–190
systematic inflammation, 13

technology, 86
television, 218
temazepam (Restoril), 74
tension, 28, 58
releasing emotional, 72–74
testosterone, 121, 122
theta waves, 10
timeless genes, 85–86
Tim protein, 85
tonsils, 207, 210
topiramate, 160
train accidents, 112, 113
transient insomnia, 51, 58–60
traumatic brain injury (TBI), 188
triazolam (Halcion), 74
type 2 diabetes, 13, 118–119

ulcers, 13
upper airway, 114, 115
URGE, 49–50
urination, nighttime, 121
uvolopalatopharyngoplasty
(UPPP), 125

Valium, 80
varicose veins, 49–50
veterans
paradoxical sleep in, 76–77
PTSD in, 123, 184–185, 190–191,
194–196
video polysomnogram, 174
violent behaviors, 169, 174, 177

violent dreams, 175–176
violent sleepwalking episodes,
   139–140

wakefulness-promoting agents,
   106
warm baths, 25
Watch-PAT, 178
weight gain, 12
weight loss, 119, 124, 131
Wellbutrin, 45

women
   insomnia and, 66–67
   with sleep apnea, 120, 122–123
worrying, 26–28

yellow color, 23

zietgebers, 91, 94, 98
zolpidem (Ambien), 75, 144, 156,
   165, 166
Zyprexa (olanzapine), 164

About the Author

Robert S. Rosenberg, DO, FCCP, is the medical director of the Sleep Disorders Center of Prescott Valley, Arizona, a sleep medicine consultant for Mountain Heart Health Services in Flagstaff, Arizona, and is board certified in sleep medicine, pulmonary medicine, and internal medicine. He is a contributing sleep expert blogger at EverydayHealth.com and his advice has appeared in *O, The Oprah Magazine, Women's Health, Prevention, Ladies' Home Journal,* and *Parenting,* among others. He lives in Prescott, Arizona.

www.AnswersForSleep.com